Intermittent Fasting for Women Over 50

The Essential Guide to Lose Weight, Increase Your Energy, Unlock Your Metabolism, and Detox Your Body for a Lasting Lifestyle

Romy Daysi Garner

Table of Contents

Introduction 1
Chapter 1: What Is Intermittent fasting? 3
   Basics of Intermittent Fasting..3
   Can Intermittent Fasting Be Related To Weight Loss? ..5
   Debunking Myths Related to Intermittent Fasting 8
      #1: Fasting will reduce your metabolic rate............... 8
      #2: You need to stay away from water consumption at the time of fasting 9
      #3: It is not possible to gain muscle at the time of fasting 9
      #4: Fasting will make you overindulge 10
      #5: It can be attempted by everyone 10
Chapter 2: All You Need to Know About Intermittent Fasting 12
   How Does Intermittent Fasting Affect Your Hormones and Cells? 13
   A Powerful Tool for Losing Weight................................... 15
   Makes Your Lifestyle Simpler and Healthier 15
   Should Women Opt for Fasting? 16
   Side Effects and Risks... 17
      Brain fog or fatigue 17
      Feeling irritated..18
      Food obsessions 18
      Low level of blood sugar 19
      Alteration in the menstrual cycle 19
      Loss of hair 20
      Constipation 21
      Disturbance of sleep.. 21

Unhealthy diet..22
Mood swings 23
Chapter 3: Intermittent Fasting and Its Types ... 24
Seven Ways of Doing Intermittent Fasting...................25
12 hours fasting...25
16:8 fasting..26
5:2 diet..27
Alternate day fasting.................................29
Eat stop eat..30
The warrior diet 31
Meal skipping...33
Tips to Maintain Intermittent Fasting 34
Chapter 4: Benefits of Intermittent Fasting 37
It Helps In Changing the Function of Genes, Cells, and Hormones 37
It Can Help In Losing Belly Fat and Weight..................38
It Helps In the Reduction of Insulin Resistance and Also Lowers the Risk of Type 2 Diabetes 39
It Can Help In the Reduction of Oxidative Stress Along With Inflammation..40
It Is Beneficial for Heart Health 41
It Induces Several Processes of Cell Repair 41
It Helps In the Prevention of Cancer............................42
It Is Good for the Brain Functioning.............................42
It Helps In the Prevention of Alzheimer's Disease........43
It Helps In Enhancing Your Lifespan............................43
Chapter 5: Tips and Tricks for Getting Started With Intermittent Fasting......................................45
Start Small 45
Determining Your Goals 46
Timing the Fast for Social Reasons 46
Taking Water for Breakfast...47
Choosing Coffee or Tea 47

- Having a Cheat Day 48
- Knowing the Difference Between Wanting to Eat and Need to Eat 48
- Eating When Needed 49
- Breaking the Fast Steadily and Slowly 50
- Stay Away From Overeating 50
- Maintaining Balanced Meals 51
- Playing Around With Various Time Periods 51
- Steering Clear of 24-Hour Fasts 52
- Adapting Your Routine of Workout 53
- Keeping Track of the Journey 53
- Listening to the Body 54

Chapter 6: List of Foods and Drinks 55
- Food 55
  - Berries 55
  - Nuts 56
  - Grains 56
  - Lentils 57
  - Seitan 57
  - Papaya 58
  - Avocado 59
  - Potato 59
  - Fish 60
  - Hummus 60
  - Cruciferous Vegetables 61
- Drinks 62
  - Water 62
  - Coffee 63
  - Tea 63
  - Apple cider vinegar 64

Chapter 7: Intermittent Fasting and Its Secrets .. 66
- Tea: The Best Companion of Intermittent Fasting 66
- Water and Its Benefits 68

Opt for Aromatherapy 69
Get Better Sleep 69

Chapter 8: Salad Recipes 70
Walnut Cranberry Chicken Salad 70
Asparagus Balsamic Quinoa Salad and Baked Tofu 72
Kale Salad 74
Chicken Salad 76
Arugula Strawberry Salad With Balsamic Vinaigrette
.... 77
Shrimp Caesar Salad 79
Broccoli Salad 81
Roasted Beet and Blood Orange Salad 83
Spinach Salad 85
Buckwheat Salad 87

Chapter 9: Meat Recipes 89
Mediterranean-Style Chicken Breast and Avocado
Tapenade 89
Veggie Cheesy Chicken Salad Sandwich 91
Brussel Sprouts and Chicken 93
Easy Beef Steak With Hollandaise Sauce and Grilled
Asparagus 94
Chimichurri Chicken Tray Bake 96
Capsicum and Cheese Stuffed Meatloaf 98
Steak Taco Bowl 101
Caprese Chicken Bowl 103

Chapter 10: Seafood Recipes 105
Cod Loin With Browned Butter and Horseradish .. 105
Creamy Fish Casserole 107
Sesame Crusted Salmon and Cauli-Rice 109
Crab Zucchini Melts 112
Seared Salmon With Lemony Sauce 114
Smoked Mussels Casserole 116
Harissa Shrimp Skewers 118

Chapter 11: Activities to Opt For 120
   Physical Activities to Enhance the Effectivity of
   Intermittent Fasting 120
   Benefits of Exercising While Practicing Intermittent
   Fasting 123
   Extent of Exercises for Weight Loss While Practicing
   Intermittent Fasting 124
   How to Get Started With a Proper Workout Session
   While Fasting? 125
      Paying attention to timing 125
      Having proper meals 126
      Deciding the type of exercise based on macros 126
   Working Out Safely At the Time of Fasting 127

Chapter 12: Five Commonly Made Mistakes 129
   Jumping Into Intermittent Fasting Too Fast 130
   Choosing the Wrong Plan 131
   Consuming Excessive Food During the Eating Window
   132
   Not Having Enough During The Eating Period 132
   Ignoring "What" Because of "When" 133

Chapter 13: Tips to Manage Menopause 135
   Having Enough Veggies and Fruits 136
   Consumption of Enough Water 137
   Having Food Items Rich In Calcium and Vitamin D .. 137
   Maintaining Healthy Body Weight 139
   Daily Workouts 139
   Keeping Distance From Trigger Foods 140
   Consuming Food Items Rich In Protein 141
   Staying Away From Skipping Meals 141
   No Smoking 142
   Having Food Items Rich In Phytoestrogen 142
   Staying Away From Processed and Refined Sugar Food
   Items 143

Dealing With Symptoms 143
   Controlling night sweats... 144
   Urinary problems... 144
   Anxiety and depression 145
   Mood swings 145

Chapter 14: Exercises for Losing Weight........... 147
Walking 147
Running or Jogging.. 148
Cycling.. 149
Weight Training.. 150
Interval Training 150
Swimming 151

Chapter 15: Intermittent Fasting and Its Effects In Slowing Down Aging 153
Causes of Aging.. 153
Anti-Aging Properties of Intermittent Fasting 161
Intermittent Fasting and Skin Health........................ 162

Conclusion 164

Introduction

Congratulations on purchasing *Intermittent Fasting for Women Over 50,* and thank you for doing so.

The chapters that you will find in this guidebook will discuss in detail every aspect of intermittent fasting that you need to know for getting started. Intermittent fasting is not like any other modern-day diet plan. It concentrates on the time of consumption of food instead of the various types of food that you consume. Intermittent fasting comes along with an array of options that you can choose from. It will not be that tough for you to adjust your lifestyle with the fasting schedule. You will get to know every possible detail about intermittent fasting in this book – what to consume and what to not, benefits, how to get started, and many other things.

The information included in this guidebook is a comprehensive approach for making intermittent fasting an easy thing, specifically for women who are over the age mark of 50 years. The fasting plans of intermittent fasting differ a bit for men and women. For example, the nutritional needs of men and women will not be the same. In simple terms, this is an all-in-one guidebook that will help you in every possible step to get started with intermittent fasting.

There are plenty of books on this subject on the market, thanks again for choosing this one! Every effort was made to ensure it is full of as much useful information as possible, please enjoy!

Chapter 1: What Is Intermittent fasting?

Intermittent fasting is a pattern of eating where you will have to properly manage your schedule of eating to get the most out of it. It cannot be regarded as a diet that will make some changes in the type of food that you consume; however, it aims for managing the time of eating. We will discuss the basics of intermittent fasting in detail in this chapter.

Basics of Intermittent Fasting

Intermittent fasting is not like regular fasting, where you have to stay without having any kind of food for one whole day or for several days. There is a huge line that exists between starvation and fasting, and there exists 'control.' Starvation is all about keeping the body away from all types of food items for a long time. On the other hand, fasting involves intentional avoidance of consumption of food for either spiritual, health, or other reasons. It is generally opted by all those individuals who are not underweight and also comes with enough fat stored to live without consumption of food. When done in the correct way, it will never result in death or any kind of suffering. Food will be readily available for you, but you will try not to have them. You can opt for the same for any period of time – three to four hours to even a couple of days.

You can also extend the same for a whole week when presented with medical supervision. Any possible time when you are not having any kind of food, you are intermittently fasting. For example, you might decide not to have anything between your breakfast and dinner for one day. It comes down to an approximate period of twelve hours. So, you can think of intermittent fasting as a natural part of your daily life. Intermittent fasting involves a certain pattern of food consumption that cycles between alternate periods of fasting and eating. The main goal of intermittent fasting is to pay close attention to the time of food consumption without paying much attention to the food types you opt for. So, you can regard intermittent fasting as not any other conventional plan of diet in this context; however, a definite pattern of eating.

The most common patterns of intermittent fasting involve fasting for sixteen hours and twenty-four hours, twice every week. Fasting has always been known as a famous practice that can also be recorded in the entire course of human evolution. People from the past did not have the provision of refrigerators, supermarkets, or stored food. So, they opted for fasting for long time periods as they didn't have anything to eat. It can be said that human beings evolved with the power of functioning properly without eating anything for long periods of time. Also, fasting is often considered a more natural thing than eating 3 – 4 meals every day. Let us start by taking into consideration the common term 'breakfast.' It is considered to be the meal that helps in breaking the all-night fast that we all do regularly. Intermittent fasting is nothing more or unusual and is a part of our normal lives.

Can Intermittent Fasting Be Related To Weight Loss?

As you opt for intermittent fasting, it will permit the body to use up all the stored forms of energy by burning the excess stored fat. It is quite important to understand that human beings have evolved in a way where they can fast for several time periods, a few hours, or even a day, without showcasing or facing any form of adverse health issue. When you make up your mind not to have anything, your body will begin the mechanism of using up stored body fat for the generation of energy. When you consume food, a huge amount of food energy is ingested that needs to be used by the body immediately. Some part of this food energy gets stored for later usage as fat. The hormone that plays the most important part in the storage of food energy is insulin. When you keep consuming food, the insulin level in your body also goes up.

It provides help in the storage of extra energy in two ways. Carbs get broken down into glucose or sugar units that get associated for creating long glycogen chains. It is stored in the liver muscles. But the overall storage space for carbs is quite limited. After a certain level is reached, the liver will start turning extra glucose into body fat. The entire process is termed de-novo lipogenesis. One portion of the newly generated fat will get stored in your liver. However, a major portion of the same will get exported to the other deposits of fat in your body. Indeed, the entire process might feel a bit complicated, but there is no form of limit to the overall amount of fat that can be produced. Thus, there are two systems of storing food energy in our bodies. The first system is easily accessible; however, it comes with very limited storage – glycogen. The second system is quite tough to be accessed; however, it comes with infinite storage – body fat.

The entire process will begin running in the reverse direction when you think not to consume food. The insulin level will fall and will make the body aware of starting with the process of burning the stored food energy as there is no energy supply from food items as you fast. The blood glucose level is also most likely to fall. So, the body will now try to pull out glucose right from the storage to produce the required energy. The human body typically exists in two proper states – the fed state and the fasted state. Human beings are either storing food energy or are burning energy from the storage. If you decide to start having food the very moment you wake up from sleep and keep doing the same until you again go back to sleep at night, you are most likely to spend most of your time in the fed state.

With time, you will slowly start gaining weight as you do not let the body burn out or use the energy that is saved in storage. In order to lose weight or to restore balance, you will have to concentrate on enhancing the time that you dedicate to burn the stored form of energy. It is the time when intermittent fasting comes into action. It will permit the body to start using the food energy that is stored in the body. As you try to concentrate on intermittent fasting for certain hours or a day, your body will soon feel deprived of the necessary energy for proper functioning. That is when the body will begin burning the fat stored in the body for energy production.

Debunking Myths Related to Intermittent Fasting

Intermittent fasting can be considered a hot topic today, and that is why there is a wide range of myths that can be found everywhere. We will debunk some of the basic myths related to intermittent fasting in this chapter.

#1: Fasting will reduce your metabolic rate

There are people who tend to worry that fasting will lower their rate of resting metabolism. The main concern is that as you start consuming food normally again, you are most likely to put on weight. All of this is very common in all those diets that focus on calorie restriction. Your body's metabolism will adapt itself to the intake of low energy, and it can easily stay as it is for years. Well, the same is not the case with intermittent fasting. In a study from the year 2005 that was published in the Clinical Nutrition Journal, people who were non-obese opted for alternate-day fasting and also had a normal rate of metabolism for three weeks; everything while burning more amount of fat.

#2: *You need to stay away from water consumption at the time of fasting*

There are a number of religious fasts where it is needed to opt for water and food restriction. In fact, there are several claims that no-water fasts are the best ones for human health. But as fasting comes with a diuretic effect, water restriction might result in excessive dehydration. That is the reason why doctors tend to pay more attention to the intake of fluids while supervising patients who opt for therapeutic fasts. You need to drink water while fasting to prevent dehydration and also to maintain fasting in the best way possible.

#3: *It is not possible to gain muscle at the time of fasting*

For the majority of people, fasting does not seem like a great way of building muscle. After all, you will always need protein shakes, right? Well, you definitely need protein; however, that is not needed 24*7. In a study from the year 2019, active women who opted for the 16/8 mode of fasting gained an equal percentage of muscle along with strength as all those women who were on a conventional eating schedule. Here is the main thing – your body will have to work hard to preserve the muscles at the time of scarcity. As you fast, your body turns to body fat for all the energy requirements. Try to think in this way: if human beings burned muscles at the time of fasting, our ancestors would have been excessively weak for hunting.

#4: Fasting will make you overindulge

After getting done with a period of fasting, you will definitely feel hungry. Many people tend to assume that this hunger will result in subsequent overeating. The evidence for this does not tend to support this myth. The majority of studies related to fasting permits participants to consume food as much as they want to – it is known as ad libitum feeding. They consume their fill and still lose a considerable amount of weight. In fact, you will be eating less on the majority of intermittent fasting protocols. The mild calorie limitation will help in the promotion of weight loss without even slowing down your metabolic rate.

#5: It can be attempted by everyone

Intermittent fasting is quite a trending topic now. In some of the cases, it is also marketed as being useful for people of all age groups.

Although fasting is a healthy and safe option for the majority of people, there are certain groups that need to stay away from the same such as pregnant women, children, and underweight people. Such groups need to consume more food and should not try to restrict food consumption. The overall risk of nutrient deficiency can easily outweigh any potential benefit of fasting. All those who suffer from a high level of blood sugar are also needed to move ahead with caution.

Chapter 2: All You Need to Know About Intermittent Fasting

As you eat, your body will spend the next couple of hours digesting the same where it gets broken down into several molecules in order to assist easy absorption into the stream of blood. It ultimately helps in easing the uptake of nutrients by the cells. The body needs about five hours to break down several macronutrients to the energy molecules. Of all the molecules, glucose is the one that can get absorbed into the bloodstream easily. The body is quite fast in absorbing glucose for transporting the same to the various parts of the body. When glucose enters the bloodstream, the body responds to the same by secreting insulin, whose main function is to help the cells to absorb glucose. It is done by sending signals to the body cells for opening up and taking up the glucose. If you had carbs in your meals, it is something that is required by the cells. The excess of the same gets channeled to the liver for conversion into glycogen with the help of insulin.

However, the glycogen storage capacity is limited. When the stores get filled, the extra glucose gets converted into glycerol and fatty acids. The body takes about eight to twelve hours from the last meal to utilize the available glucose in the bloodstream. When you do not consume any kind of food item rich in calories for a minimum of fourteen hours, the energy storage process will start going in the opposite direction. In simple terms, the body will enter a mode of burning energy. If you want to opt for effective weight loss, you will have to allow your body to stay without any kind of food rich in calories for a minimum of 14 hours. It is what the program of intermittent fasting seeks to attain – to get you in a position of metabolism where your body is forced to use up all the stored energy as this will turn on the energy-burning mechanism of the body.

How Does Intermittent Fasting Affect Your Hormones and Cells?

When you start fasting, there are a couple of things that happen in the body, both on the molecular and cellular levels. For instance, your body starts adjusting the levels of hormones to make the stored body fat even more accessible. The body cells also start essential processes of repairing and also alters the genetic expressions. Let's have a look at some of the changes that take place in the body as you fast.

- **HGH or human growth hormone:** The level of human growth hormone tends to go up, increasing to about five-fold. It provides various benefits for muscle gain and fat loss, naming a few.

- **Cellular repair:** While your body is in a fasted state, your cells will start the processes of cell repair. It involves autophagy, where the cells remove and digest the dysfunctional and old proteins that tend to pile up inside the cells.

- **Insulin:** Sensitivity to insulin enhances, and the level of insulin also drops drastically. Having a lower level of insulin will make stored fat even more accessible.

- **Genetic expression:** There are various changes in the functioning of genes that are related to protection against disease along with longevity.

All such changes in cell functioning, hormone levels, and genetic expression are responsible for the benefits of intermittent fasting.

A Powerful Tool for Losing Weight

Weight loss is the primary reason why the majority of people opt for intermittent fasting. As you opt for eating fewer meals, intermittent fasting will result in an automatic reduction in the intake of calories. Also, intermittent fasting alters the levels of hormones, as we already know, for facilitating weight loss. Besides increasing the levels of growth hormone and lowering the levels of insulin, intermittent fasting also enhances the release of the hormone norepinephrine, which is responsible for burning fat. Owing to the hormonal changes, fasting for the short-term can help in enhancing your rate of metabolism by about 3.5% - 13%. By making you eat few and burn more amount of calories, the process of intermittent fasting results in weight loss by altering both sides of the calorie equation.

Makes Your Lifestyle Simpler and Healthier

Eating healthy is a simple thing to do; however, it might be quite hard to maintain the same. The biggest obstacle that you might face while trying to eat healthy is to plan out and cook all your healthy meals. Intermittent will make everything even simpler for you, as you will not need to cook or plan for your meals. Just for this reason, intermittent fasting is quite popular among all those people who are too busy with their lives as it helps in enhancing your health, besides making your life simpler.

Should Women Opt for Fasting?

There are some pieces of evidence that indicate that intermittent fasting might not be that useful for women in comparison to men. For instance, in a study, it improved sensitivity to insulin in men; however, it worsened the level of blood sugar in women. Although enough human studies on intermittent fasting are not much available, some studies in female rats showed that intermittent fasting can make them masculinized, emaciated, infertile, and might also result in missing cycles. There are also various reports related to women whose menstrual period just stopped as they started with intermittent fasting and also went back to the normal state as they resumed their old pattern of eating. For all such reasons, women are needed to be extra careful while getting started with intermittent fasting. They will have to follow some other guidelines, such as practicing the program and then immediately stopping in case there is some kind of problem, such as amenorrhea or the absence of menstruation. In case you have some kind of issues related to fertility, or if you are trying to conceive, it will be better for you if you can consider holding off on the program of intermittent fasting at the moment.

Side Effects and Risks

When it comes to intermittent fasting, there are various types of risks and side effects related to the same. There are some red flags that you will need to be careful of.

Brain fog or fatigue

Have you ever seen yourself yawning right in the morning, only to realize that you never had your breakfast? As not having your breakfast is a typical way of opting for intermittent fasting, understanding that you are extremely tired daily, or just keep making some mistakes as you are experiencing brain fog is a clear sign that you do not have the right foods during your non-fasting hours. It might also be the case that fasting is not properly fitting your lifestyle. You will have to pay attention to what you are feeding your body with. You can have anything while being on intermittent fasting. However, you will still have to provide your body with good food that can make you feel strong and healthy. So, it can be said that intermittent fasting might result in fatigue or brain fog.

Feeling irritated

As you try to stay without food, feeling grumpy, irritable, and grouchy are some of the feelings that you will surely experience. All such feelings come with the inability to not consume any kind of food when your body is signaling you that you are hungry. Teaching your body to stay without food for about 12 – 16 hours will need some practice. In fact, the bodies of some people might not be happy ever with consuming food within a constricted window. Theoretically, if you have enough protein in any of your meals, you should not be starving early in the morning. However, in case you keep starving on a daily basis in the morning, then you might have to make some adjustments during your periods of calorie consumption to prevent crankiness. There are people for whom not consuming food for a long time might not be the ideal thing. So, you will have to consider this before you start with the same.

Food obsessions

As you try to be on some kind of restrictive diet, it can easily affect your relationship with food.

While there are people who actually like the rigidity that comes with intermittent fasting, other people might find themselves concentrating excessively on when they can consume food and the number of calories that they are getting. Spending a great amount of time thinking about the quantity or quality of food on a regular basis might result in a type of eating disorder termed orthorexia. Having orthorexia indicates that you pay so much attention to healthful or correct eating that it results in having some kind of detrimental effect on your well-being.

Low level of blood sugar

If you are experiencing headaches, nausea, or dizziness persistently while practicing intermittent fasting, it is a red flag that the fasting process is lowering your level of blood sugar. For this very reason, diabetics need to stay away from any kind of fasting diet. In fact, intermittent fasting might turn you into being hypoglycemic, a serious condition for anyone suffering from thyroid or insulin problems.

Alteration in the menstrual cycle

Women who tend to lose a great amount of weight or are not getting the required number of calories every day might suffer from slowing down of their menstrual cycle or even complete stoppage of the same. Women having low body weight are very much prone to a condition termed amenorrhea or temporary absence of menstruation, which we have already discussed before. Experiencing a sudden loss of weight or being underweight might result in disruption of the typical hormone cycle and lead to missed cycles. So, while you might be glad of the way in which intermittent fasting helped you lose weight, you might also be depriving the body of the required calories that are needed for functioning.

Loss of hair

Opting for a fasting diet can result in hair loss. Is this even true? Well, yes, it is. Sudden reduction of weight or lack of necessary nutrients, specifically B vitamins and protein, can result in hair loss. An essential point that you should always keep in mind – although intermittent fasting does not result in loss of nutrients, it makes it harder to consume a properly balanced diet as your body is cramming for consuming food worth a whole day within a few hours only. In case you find out that you have excessive hair loss daily, you might need to reevaluate the nutritional content of the daily meals and also consult with your doctor to make sure whether intermittent fasting is a good choice for you or not.

Constipation

Any form of diet might result in an upset stomach in case you fail to get enough vitamins, fluids, fiber, or protein. It is an easy thing for the majority of people to just forget to drink enough water at the time of fasting. However, opting for a fast of 16 hours without trying to have enough water is a great recipe for gastrointestinal disaster. So, if you have just started with the program of intermittent fasting and do not seem to have regular bowel movements, it might be time to hit a pause on the plan and consult a nutritionist for the same to find out what is happening exactly.

Disturbance of sleep

There are people who reported having improved patterns of sleep after getting started with intermittent fasting. It might be because of the way intermittent fasting helps in curbing the habits of late-night snacking, which can easily make it a tough thing for you to fall asleep as your stomach will be busy digesting your 10 p.m. food. But there is some recent research that points out the exact opposite. A review from the year 2018 in the Nature and Science of Sleep journal points out that intermittent fasting points out that diurnal intermittent fasting results in a decrease of REM or rapid-eye-movement sleep. Having enough REM sleep is often linked with all forms of health benefits, along with better memory, concentration, and also cognitive processing.

In case you come to find out that you are having difficulty falling asleep or staying asleep after you started with the program of intermittent fasting, hit a pause once again and consult an expert to ensure that it is not harming your health.

Unhealthy diet

Even if intermittent fasting does not tend to trigger some serious disorders, such as orthorexia, it could still breed in some unhealthy habits of eating. Besides not getting enough nutrition, you might also find yourself making messy nutritious choices at the time of eating. The primary concern is staying away from the habit of binge-eating as you might get so hungry during the fasting hours that you might just consume 5,000 calories at once. If you find this similar to you, it will be better for you to work in collaboration with a dietician to structure a plan for you that will not force you to constrict the eating hours and just concentrate on providing your body with the necessary nutrients.

Mood swings

It would sound weird if you didn't ever experience any form of moodiness at the time of practicing intermittent fasting, or at least while starting with the same. While there are people who can feel some great boost of motivation or energy once they start with the program of fasting, it is also essential to keep in mind that it is still a diet of restrictive nature. Feeling the obligation to follow the same might lead to negative effects on your overall mood, specifically if you get isolated from family and friends because of your diet limitations. If you start feeling anxious, discouraged, or down regarding intermittent fasting, it will be better for you to stop and just get in touch with a dietician. They might help you in designing a proper schedule of fasting that will better suit your body and mind.

Chapter 3: Intermittent Fasting and Its Types

When it comes to intermittent fasting, there are several ways of doing the same. The methods tend to vary in the total hours of fasting or number of days besides the allowances of calories. Intermittent fasting is all about partially or entirely abstaining yourself from consuming any kind of food for a specific period of time, right before you start eating again on your regular form. There are studies that determine the various types of benefits of intermittent fasting, like loss of weight, better health, enhanced longevity, and many others. It is also said that it an easier thing to maintain intermittent fasting than the other types of traditional diet plans that involve restriction of calories. The experience of each person with intermittent fasting is completely different, and the different styles of doing the same will suit different people. We will discuss the most popular types of intermittent fasting in this chapter, along with certain tips that will help you to maintain the diet.

Seven Ways of Doing Intermittent Fasting

There are various ways in which intermittent fasting can be done, and every individual will prefer different styles.

12 hours fasting

The schedule of this form of fasting is regarded to be the easiest of all, least painful, and is also a more natural way of fasting. If you have your last meal at 8 p.m., then you cannot have your next meal until 8 a.m. in the morning. If you have some kind of late snack at 10 p.m., then you will not be able to have your next meal until 10 a.m. in the morning. The aim is to fast for a period of twelve hours straight. You can also do the exact opposite – have your breakfast at 8 a.m. in the morning and then opt for the next meal at 8 p.m. in the evening. The method of 12 hours fasting is quite flexible and is also a great option for balancing the metabolism and hormones of women. If you are thinking of starting with intermittent fasting, then this option might be the easiest one for you to start with and get a hold of the fasting program.

According to some studies, if you try to fast for about 10 – 16 hours, it can result in turning the fat stores of your body into useful energy, which results in the release of ketones into your bloodstream. It can easily result in weight loss. The fasting window in this type of intermittent fasting is relatively small, where the majority of the fasting takes place at the time of sleeping. You will also be able to have the same number of calories every day.

16:8 fasting

In this method of intermittent fasting, you will have to consume all your meals within a window of eight hours and then opt for fasting for the remaining sixteen hours. Within the eating window of eight hours, it is always suggested to arrange about 2 – 3 meals. In simple terms, you will have to stop consumption of food right after having your dinner and then skip your breakfast as well the next morning. For instance, if you tend to finish your last meal by 8 p.m. in the evening, then you will not have any other food until 12 p.m. the next day. It will establish the 16:8 fasting method. For all those individuals who tend to get hungry early in the morning, the schedule of the 16:8 method might turn out to be a bit problematic for them to embrace. Well, you can push back your morning window by half an hour every day until you get comfortable waiting till 12 p.m. to start your eating window of eight hours.

You can opt for having coffee, water, or other types of drinks that come with no form of calories during the window of fasting. It will help in reducing the hunger feeling and will also make the transition a lot easy for you. It is always recommended to opt for wholesome and healthy food during the eating window. The 16:8 method might turn out to be useful for someone who has already tried the 12 hours fasting and hasn't seen benefits of any kind. In a study involving mice, it was found that limiting the window of feeding to eight hours helped in protecting them from inflammation, obesity, liver disease, and also diabetes.

5:2 diet

In the method of 5:2 diet, you will have limited calories for two days a week and five days of normal eating. On the days of limited calories, it is suggested for women to have about 500 calories and 600 calories for men. You will have to start by eating normally for five days every week. By normal eating, we mean to eat a healthy and clean diet that is composed of healthy meats, whole foods, and other necessary nutrient-rich food items. For the two days of fasting, you can have either one proper meal of 500 calories or two small meals of 250 calories each. You can consume coffee, water, and other calorie-free drinks at the time of fasting. Limiting your calorie intake for two days will make it hard for you to create sustainable meals. You will have to make sure that you follow whole food and a healthy diet during the eating window of five days. You will have to make a proper balance between raw veggies and fruits that will help the stomach to stay full for a longer time.

You can pair fiver with your meals, like oatmeal, and plant-based proteins such as hemp seeds and flaxseeds. Generally, people separate their days of fasting into one week. For instance, you can fast on Monday and Thursday and keep eating normally for the rest of the days. You will have to keep a minimum of one non-fasting day in between the days of fasting. A limited amount of research can be found for the 5:2 diet plan, which is also termed the Fast diet. A study involving 108 obese or overweight women found that calorie restriction for two days in a week and consistent calorie restriction both resulted in a similar kind of weight loss. The participants of the diet also had reduced levels of insulin along with improved sensitivity to insulin.

A small-sized study was conducted to look at the effects of this style of fasting in 23 obese women. Over the course of their menstrual cycle, the participants lost about 4.8% of their body weight and 8% of their total body fat. But the measurements went back to normal for the majority of women right after five days of eating normally.

Alternate day fasting

It is an approach to intermittent fasting. The main idea of this fasting method is to fast for one day and then eat normally the next day. In this way, you will only need to restrict what you consume half of the time. On the days of fasting, you can have as many calorie-free drinks as you want, like unsweetened coffee, water, or tea. If you are willing to opt for this method, you will be permitted to consume about 500 calories on the days of fasting, or about 20% - 25% of your total requirement of energy. The weight loss and health benefits tend to be the same if you try to consume the fasting-day calories at the time of lunch or dinner or as several small meals during the course of the day. There are people who find this approach of fasting much easier than any other form of diet.

The effects of alternate-day fasting on hunger are actually consistent. There are studies that show that hunger ultimately decreases during the days of fasting, while for some, it remains unchanged.

But it is agreed by all forms of research that it is an easier thing to be on 500 calories on the days of fasting than full fasts. Another important factor that you should keep in mind is compensatory hunger. It is common in the majority of traditional calorie restriction diets. Compensatory hunger is the increased levels of hunger resulting from the restriction of calories, which make people eat more than they should when they are permitted to eat again.

__Eat stop eat__

It is a unique approach to the practice of intermittent fasting that is characterized by the inclusion of two fasting days that are not consecutive every week. Implementation of this form of intermittent is pretty straightforward. You will have to select one or two non-consecutive days every week during which you will not eat anything and fast for an overall 24-hour period. For the rest of the five to six days every week, you can keep eating freely. However, it is always suggested to opt for sensible food choices and also avoid consumption of more food than the body requires. For example, if you have decided to fast from 9 a.m. Wednesday until 9 a.m. Thursday, you will have to ensure that you have one proper meal before 9 a.m. on Wednesday. The next meal that you will have will be after 9 a.m. on Thursday. In this way, you will ensure that you fast for an overall period of 24 hours.

While you practice this form of intermittent fasting, you will have to make sure that you opt for proper hydration as well. You will have to get back to your normal patterns of eating on the non-fasting days. Consuming food in this manner will help in the reduction of an individual's overall calorie intake; however, it does not restrict any kind of specific food that one consumes. Fasting for 24 hours straight might turn out to be challenging and might also result in headache, irritability, or fatigue. Make sure you get experienced with 12 hours or 16 hours of fasting first before you opt for this method.

__The warrior diet__

The warrior diet is considered a type of intermittent fasting, a term that involves eating patterns with periods of reduced intake of calories over a specified period. The diet is completely based on the patterns of eating of the ancient warriors who had the habit of eating little during the day and then feasting at night. All those who opt for this form of intermittent fasting undereat for about twenty hours every day and then eat as much as food desired during the night. During the fasting window of twenty hours, you can have small amounts of dairy items, boiled eggs, raw veggies, and fruits, along with some low-calorie drinks. After the period of twenty hours, you can binge on any kind of food that you want to within the eating window of four hours. But healthy, organic, and unprocessed food choices are generally encouraged. Anyone who is thinking of starting with the warrior diet needs to follow a plan for three weeks.

The first week or the first phase is the detox phase. During the twenty hours of fasting period for the first week, you will have to undereat and have only clear broth, vegetable juices, boiled egg, yogurt, and vegetables. During the period of overeating, you can have a salad with vinegar and oil dressing, followed by some plant proteins, cheese, cooked veggies, and wheat-free whole grains. The second week or the second phase is known as the high-fat phase. The undereating phase will be the same as that of the first week. During the eating period, you can have salad, lean animal protein, cooked veggies, and nuts. No form of starch or grains is allowed during the second phase. The third week or third phase is the concluding fat loss phase. In this phase, you will have to cycle between periods of high protein and high carb intake.

- One to two days high in carbs
- One to two days low in carbs and high in protein
- One to two days high in carbs
- One to two days low in carbs and high in protein

On the days of high-carb, you will follow the same undereating schedule. During the eating window, you can have salad, cooked veggies, a little portion of animal protein, and one primary carb like potatoes, corn, barley, oats, or pasta. On the days of high protein and low protein, the undereating phase will be the same. During the eating period, you can have salad, with eight to sixteen ounces of animal protein, along with some non-starchy cooked veggies.

Meal skipping

You are not required to follow a detailed and structured plan of intermittent fasting for reaping all of its benefits. Another great option is to simply skip your meals timely, like when you do not feel like having anything or when you are too busy to eat. It is actually a myth that human beings need to eat after every few hours, or else they will lose muscle or hit starvation mode. Our bodies are equipped properly for handling long periods of no food. So, you can easily skip one or two meals daily. When you do not feel hungry one day, try skipping breakfast, and just opt for a healthy lunch and dinner. When you are traveling somewhere and cannot get your hands on any kind of food to eat, opt for a short fast. Intentionally skipping one or two meals when you feel like doing so is a spontaneous form of doing intermittent fasting.

Meal skipping is considered to be the most successful form of intermittent fasting where people can monitor and also respond to the signals of their body hunger.

Tips to Maintain Intermittent Fasting

It might be challenging for some people to properly stick to a program of intermittent fasting. But there are tips that can help you to be on track and also maximize the positive sides of intermittent fasting. Let's have a look at them.

- Staying hydrated is very important. Try to have lots of water and other drinks that are free from calories, like herbal teas, during the course of the day.

- Try to avoid obsessing over foods. Give your best to plan a number of distractions on the days of fasting in order to stay away from thinking about food, like opting for a movie or getting busy with some paperwork.

- You will have to relax and rest. Try to stay away from all sorts of strenuous jobs on the days of fasting; however, you can opt for light exercises like yoga.

- Try to make every calorie count. If the plan that you chose permits some calories at the time of fasting, choose some nutrient-rich food items that come with a high percentage of fiber, protein, healthy fats.

- Opt for food items that come with high volume. You will have to choose filling yet low-calorie food items, like raw veggies, fruits, popcorn, and many others.

- You can improve the taste of your foods without even enhancing the calories. Season your meals generously with herbs, spices, vinegar, and garlic. All these food items come with a low calorific value and can also make your food rich in flavor, which can easily help in reducing the feeling of hunger.

- You will have to choose nutrient-dense food items after the period of fasting. Consuming food items that are rich in vitamins, minerals, fiber, and several other essential nutrients can help in maintaining a steady level of blood sugar and also avoid nutrient deficiencies. Following a balanced diet will also help in weight loss along with improvement of overall health.

Chapter 4: Benefits of Intermittent Fasting

Intermittent fasting is a popular topic today owing to the wide range of benefits of the program. Indeed, everything in this world comes with its own array of downsides, but in the case of intermittent fasting, the benefits can easily outnumber the downsides. The following are the benefits of intermittent fasting that you can enjoy when you follow the methods properly.

It Helps In Changing the Function of Genes, Cells, and Hormones

As you do not consume food for a while, there are several things happening inside your body. For instance, your body will start the process of cell repair and will also alter the levels of hormones for making the stored body fat more accessible for energy. Here are some of the proper changes that tend to occur in the body at the time of fasting.

- **Insulin level:** The levels of insulin significantly drops, which helps in the burning of fat.

- **Human growth hormone:** The levels of growth hormone might increase by five-fold. Higher levels of the hormone help in muscle gain and fat burning as well. It also comes with various other benefits.

- **Gene expression:** There are essential alterations in several genes along with molecules that are linked to protection against diseases and longevity.

- **Cellular repair:** The body will start various essential cell repair processes, like the removal of waste material from the cells.

A majority of the benefits of intermittent fasting are associated with all such changes in gene expression, hormones, and cell functioning.

It Can Help In Losing Belly Fat and Weight

The majority of people who opt for intermittent fasting are because of losing weight. Generally, intermittent fasting will always make you consume fewer meals. Unless you can compensate by eating more during the eating hours, you will be consuming fewer calories. Also, intermittent fasting helps in improving hormone functioning for facilitating weight loss. Lower levels of insulin increased levels of norepinephrine, and higher levels of growth hormone all help in enhancing the breakdown of body fat and use up the same for energy. For this very reason, fasting for a short time period helps in increasing the metabolic rate by about 3.5% - 13.6%, helping you to burn more calories. In simple terms, intermittent fasting can function on all sides of the equation. It helps in boosting up the rate of metabolism while reducing the total amount of food that you consume.

A study from the year 2014 revealed that you could lose about 3% - 8% of your weight within a period of 3 – 24 weeks. In fact, you can lose about 5% – 7% of your waist circumference, which is an indication of losing belly fat. Also, it has been found that intermittent fasting results in less muscle loss in comparison to the traditional types of calorie-restrictive diets.

It Helps In the Reduction of Insulin Resistance and Also Lowers the Risk of Type 2 Diabetes

Type 2 diabetes is a common problem in today's world. The main feature of type 2 diabetes is high levels of blood sugar in the context of resistance to insulin. Anything that helps in the reduction of insulin resistance can also help in lowering the levels of blood sugar and also provide protection against type 2 diabetes. Well, intermittent fasting has shown some incredible results in the reduction of insulin resistance and also an impressive reduction in the levels of blood sugar. In some studies involving human beings, fasting blood sugar was reduced by 4% - 6% while fasting insulin was reduced by 21% - 30%. A study involving diabetic rats showed that intermittent fasting could provide protection against kidney damage, which is often considered as one of the primary complications of diabetes. So, it can be said that intermittent fasting can be protective for all those people who are at risk of developing type 2 diabetes.

It Can Help In the Reduction of Oxidative Stress Along With Inflammation

Oxidative stress is one of the first steps in the direction of aging and several types of chronic diseases. It is all about unstable molecules known as free radicals, which tend to interact with other essential molecules and just damage them. There are studies that show that intermittent fasting can help in enhancing the resistance of your body to oxidative stress. Also, intermittent fasting can help in dealing with inflammation which acts as another key for all sorts of chronic diseases.

It Is Beneficial for Heart Health

Heart diseases are currently the largest killers in the world. It is known to all of us that several health markers are linked to either a decreased or increased risk of heart diseases. Intermittent fasting has proved to enhance numerous risk factors, along with blood pressure, blood triglycerides, LDL cholesterol, blood sugar levels, and inflammatory markers. But a majority of this is based on studies related to animals. The overall effects of intermittent fasting on human heart health are yet to be studied.

It Induces Several Processes of Cell Repair

As we start fasting, the body cells start the process of waste removal, which is termed autophagy. It involves breaking down the cells and then metabolization of the dysfunctional and broken proteins that can be found inside the cells. Enhanced rate of autophagy can help in providing protection against various types of diseases, along with Alzheimer's disease and cancer.

It Helps In the Prevention of Cancer

Cancer is a dangerous disease that is characterized by an uncontrollable growth of cells. Fasting has shown several benefits on metabolism that can help in reducing the risk of developing cancer. Although studies related to human beings are still needed, evidence from animal studies suggests that intermittent fasting can help in the prevention of cancer. There is also some evidence on cancer patients that showed reduced side effects of chemotherapy because of fasting.

It Is Good for the Brain Functioning

All those things that are considered to be good for the body are often for the brain too. Intermittent fasting enhances several metabolic features that are considered to be essential for the health of the brain. It includes reduced inflammation, reduced oxidative stress, and also a reduction in the levels of blood sugar along with insulin resistance. A number of studies in rats showed that intermittent fasting could enhance the growth of brand new nerve cells, which can also benefit brain functioning. It also helps in increasing the levels of the brain hormone BDNF or brain-derived neurotrophic factor. Deficiency of this hormone might result in depression along with several other brain-related problems.

It Helps In the Prevention of Alzheimer's Disease

Alzheimer's disease is known as the most common type of neurodegenerative disease in the world. There is still no proper cure available for the same, and so prevention of the disease before it shows up in the first place is a critical thing to do. A recent study in rats showed that intermittent fasting could help in delaying the onset of Alzheimer's disease or even reduce the severity. In a series of reports, an intervention of lifestyle that involved short-term fasts on a daily basis was able to improve the symptoms of Alzheimer's disease in nine out of ten patients. But still, more research based on human beings is needed to understand its overall effectiveness.

It Helps In Enhancing Your Lifespan

One of the most interesting applications of intermittent fasting might be its ability to improve lifespan. Several studies in rats showed that intermittent fasting could help in extending lifespan in the same way as constant calorie restriction. In some of the studies, the results appeared to be a bit dramatic. In one of the studies, rats that experienced fasting every alternate day lived 84% longer in comparison to the rats that were not put under the program of fasting. Provided the wide range of benefits related to metabolism and several forms of health markers, it makes complete sense that the program of intermittent fasting can help you in living a longer life besides being healthy.

Chapter 5: Tips and Tricks for Getting Started With Intermittent Fasting

Although intermittent fasting is quite simple to follow, the tips and tricks that you will find in this section will help you to get started with intermittent fasting.

Start Small

Just like every other new thing in life, if you are willing to set yourself up for success, it is quite essential to begin small with the program of intermittent fasting. So, what exactly is starting small? Well, you can begin by pushing all your meals only a little so that you can have a longer time before opting for the next meal. With time, you will reach a point where you will be able to skip a complete meal with ease. For example, in place of having your breakfast at 8 a.m., you can push it one hour ahead so that you can have your meal around 9 a.m. Then, you might not take your lunch at 1 p.m. and just push the same to 4 p.m. If you have your meals this late, you can easily take small-sized meals for your dinner or just skip the same. All of this will help in getting you accustomed to take more amount of time between all your meals, which will help you to opt for fasting for about 16 hours without any kind of problem.

With time, you will be able to increase the gap of your fasting window to get it up to 24 hours if you are ready for the same.

Determining Your Goals

Right before you opt for a suitable protocol of intermittent fasting, you will have to determine all your goals. For example, if you are willing to enhance your body composition in regards to muscle growth or fat loss, opting for 16 hours of fasting with an eating window of 8 hours every day will act as a great option for you. In order to opt for body cleansing and also for the prevention of aging, you will have to opt for a fasting period of 24 hours.

Timing the Fast for Social Reasons

For the majority of beginners, it is simpler to set an intermittent fasting window of eight hours somewhere between 9 a.m. and around 5 p.m., specifically when in social places. But opting for social programs will make you eat more meals along with more calories. It indicates that you might cheat every now and then. Also, you might feel the temptation to have something after 5 p.m. or right after you leave your workplace. An effective approach to prevent cheating is to skip breakfast along with your midmorning snack and then opt for having your meals between 12 p.m. and 8 p.m.

Taking Water for Breakfast

You can make up your mind to fast overnight until 12 p.m. and so having water in the water is a great strategy for keeping your hunger at bay during your breakfast time. You can opt for having one to two glasses of water every day after waking up so that you can revitalize your body that was dehydrated previously at the time of sleeping. In order to make sure that you actually enjoy water as your daily breakfast drink, you add lemon juice for adding extra flavor along with a pleasant smell to normal water.

Choosing Coffee or Tea

Besides water, you can opt for coffee or tea for your breakfast, provided that you do not add any kind of sweeteners like cream or sugar. You can opt for having black coffee to deal with all your hunger pangs.

Having a Cheat Day

While fixing up a cheat day can help you a lot in sticking to the program of fasting because you can have any kind of food you feel like, you can also control such kind of eating by opting for healthier options. You can have a few days where you can have high calories and just focus on having natural and unprocessed food items, like almond butter, potatoes, dark chocolate, and many others. Try to stay away from sweet food items as it might reverse all the gains in relation to your weight loss. Just concentrate on having healthy food without any kind of additives.

Knowing the Difference Between Wanting to Eat and Need to Eat

Once you get to hear that your stomach is growling, you start feeling that there is no other way of spending more hours without any kind of food. You will have to tune in to that cue of hunger. Try to ask yourself whether that hunger is actual hunger or boredom hunger. In case you are feeling bored, you will have to give your best to distract yourself with some other tasks. If you are actually hungry; however, not feeling dizzy or weak, then you can opt for a cup of war, mint tea. It is because peppermint comes with the power of reducing your appetite, or you can also opt for plain water to fill up your stomach until the next meal. Now, if you are practicing intermittent fasting for a long time and still feel excessive hunger between the eating and fasting periods, then you might have to start with some thinking.

You will have to add more calorie-dense or nutrient-dense foods during the eating window, or just consider that the current program is not the right fit for you. Adding healthy fats, like avocado, nut butter, coconut oil, and olive oil, besides proteins, at the time of eating can help you stay full for a longer period of time besides keeping you satisfied.

Eating When Needed

Generally, intense fatigue and hunger should not take place when you are on the 16:8 method of fasting. However, if you are feeling extremely lightheaded, try to listen up, as there might be some odds that the body is trying to signal you. You might have a low level of blood sugar and just require to have something. According to definition, fasting is about removing some, if not possible, to remove all, so there is nothing to beat yourself up just to break your fast with small bites. You can have some protein-rich snacks, such as a few slices of turkey breast or two boiled eggs. You can then again get back to fasting. Also, if you do not feel like fasting after having your snacks, there is no need to opt for the same.

Breaking the Fast Steadily and Slowly

After you spend some hours without any kind of food, you might turn out to be a human vacuum who is all set to suck up everything present on the plate. However, gulping down in minutes is not good for the waistline and also for your body. Instead of doing that, try to chew your food properly and just consume your food slowly to allow the same to get digested in the proper way. You will have to permit the digestive system to process the food properly. It will also provide you with a better idea of your fullness and allow you to steer clear of overeating.

Stay Away From Overeating

Only because you are done with your fast does not indicate that you can opt for a feast. Not only that excessive eating will leave you uncomfortable and bloated; however, it can also easily sabotage the goals of your weight-loss program that most likely directed you to intermittent fasting in the first place. In simple terms, it does not matter how much is present on your plate that can help you in staying full for long but what exactly is present on the plate.

Maintaining Balanced Meals

Opting for a proper mixture of fiber, protein, carbs, and healthy fats can provide you with the necessary help to shed all your excess pounds and also steer clear from excessive hunger while fasting. A great example of a balanced meal is having grilled chicken with half portion of sweet potato and some sauteed spinach with olive oil and garlic. If you are willing to opt for fruits, you will have to opt for the ones that come with a low-glycemic index, which can be slowly absorbed, metabolized, and digested, resulting in a slower and lower rise in the level of blood glucose. Having a stable level of blood sugar will help you to prevent cravings, and thus can be considered as a great key when it is about successful reduction of pounds.

Playing Around With Various Time Periods

As a beginner, the 16:8 method is generally suggested by nutritionists. However, you can have a look at your lifestyle as a whole for determining the kind of fasting method that might fit you the best. For instance, if you wake up early in the morning, you can consume food during the earlier hours, such as 9 a.m. to 5 p.m. You can then opt for fasting until the next day at 9 a.m. Keep in mind that the real beauty of intermittent fasting is that it is very flexible and amendable for fitting your schedule. Another great option is to cut yourself off earlier and then opt for breakfast later every day for growing your strength of fasting gradually. All of us naturally fast once every day, and that is at the time of sleeping. So, you might practice closing down your kitchen earlier. For instance, close your kitchen at 8 p.m. and do not opt for eating anything until your breakfast at 7 a.m. That is a natural way of opting for an 11-hour fast. You can try to move these times out slowly if you want to.

Steering Clear of 24-Hour Fasts

Experts do not recommend opting for full-day fasts as it might result in increased hunger, weakness, and also increased consumption of food. It will ultimately lead to weight gain. In case your primary goal is to lose weight, then you can try to consider the overall intake of calories and then work on the same to scale that down. It might turn out to be more beneficial than being on a fast for a long period of time. In fact, there is no form of any added benefit of 24-hours fasting in comparison to calorie restriction on a daily basis.

Adapting Your Routine of Workout

To start with this, you can surely exercise if you are opting for a fasting diet. However, if you are mindful of the types of movements that you can opt for, you will have to consider certain things. If you are willing to exercise while being in the fasted state, you will have to finish your exercise early in the morning when you generally have the maximum amount of energy. With that said, if you fail to fuel your muscles adequately, you might be at a greater risk of hurting yourself. So, you will have to opt for lower-intensity workouts, like steady-state cardio or yoga on the fasting mornings.

Keeping Track of the Journey

No matter you believe it or not, opting for a food journal can help you a lot in your fasting diet. Is it possible to have a food journal for fasting? Well, yes, you can have a food journal for fasting. While you might not be recording a great number of eats, jotting down details, such as any symptoms or emotions that you experience at the time of fasting, can provide you with the necessary help to gauge your progress.

Listening to the Body

It can be regarded as the most important point out of all. You will have to keep an eye continuously on any form of symptoms, like fatigue, dizziness, headache, irritability, difficulty concentrating, and anxiety. In case you tend to experience any of these, it will better for you to break the fast. All of these are signs that indicate that your body is slowly going into the mode of starvation, and you might need to opt for nourishment. Also, you will have to be patient with the process. It will take some time for the body to get used to the program of fasting, and you might also start feeling weaker and hungrier than usual. So, there is nothing to flip out if you tend to have all such sensations for one week or so. If all such challenges tend to last longer, and you keep experiencing symptoms, like dizziness, you might consider ditching the fasting program and opt for something else that will help in meeting your goals.

Chapter 6: List of Foods and Drinks

Intermittent fasting comes with a wide array of positive effects and benefits that can be easily reaped by opting for some suggested food items that are low in calories. The method of weight loss is not dependent on the amount of food that you consume. It concentrates on eating time. Although, there is nothing in particular regarding the kind of food items that you can consume at the time of fasting. There are some food items that will surely help in reaping the best out of the fasting program. All such food items will also help in making you feel satisfied and full for a longer time. Let us have a look at some of the foods and drinks that you can opt for to have the best results.

Food

Berries

Smoothies prepared from berries tend to form an important part of the duet plan involving intermittent fasting. For getting your daily dose of vitamin C, you can have a strawberry smoothie for your breakfast. You can also get the same amount of vitamin C by having one cup of strawberries. In fact, berries act as a great option for dealing with all forms of cravings at the time of fasting. If you are not much fond of berries, you can add some other fruits as well for making the smoothies and enhancing the taste. Opting for smoothies can give you the goodness of several food items at once. Berries also come with several other essential nutrients that can help in fulfilling your nutrient intake.

Nuts

Nuts come with the power of helping you to get rid of all sorts of body fat. It will be a good option for you if you can add some mixture of nuts in the kitchen. In fact, nuts help in enhancing longevity. Consumption of nuts can also help in the reduction of cardiovascular diseases, diabetes, and many other chronic diseases. In case you are not a big fan of nuts, you can opt for mixing the same with your smoothies.

Grains

Carbs form an important part of our lives and cannot be considered as a great enemy when it comes to the aspect of losing weight. As you will spend a huge part of your day fasting during the course of the diet, it is quite essential to give it a strategic thought regarding the ways in which you can provide the body with enough calories without feeling overly full. Although any healthy diet tries to minimize the consumption of processed food items, there might be a place and time for some items, such as bagels, whole-grain bread, and crackers. All such food items can be digested quickly and also provide easy fuel for the body. If you decide to opt for exercising on a regular basis while following intermittent fasting, all these can be a superb source of energy.

Lentils

Lentils are popular for their high content of fiber. If you can consume about half a cup of lentils on a daily basis, you can easily fulfill about 33% of the overall fiber requirement of the body in one day. In fact, lentils are also a great source of iron when needed, specifically for women who have crossed the mark of 50 years. So, if you are looking out for options to fulfill the necessary requirements of nutrition while being on the program of intermittent fasting, lentils can provide you with the needed help.

Seitan

Opting for a balanced amount of protein regularly in the diet is quite necessary for the well-being of your health. If you are not fond of animal-derived proteins, opting for alternatives is the only option left. One of the alternative sources of protein is seitan. It is often termed wheat meat. In fact, seitan is the richest protein source that can be derived from plants. Seitan is easy to bake, and you can consume the same with some sauce for fulfilling your protein requirement. Regardless of the kind of diet that you opt for, intake of protein is important for your overall well-being.

Papaya

The final hours of any fasting window will always be the most important phase as you might start feeling hungry, specifically if you are new to the program of fasting. You might end up overeating during the window of eating, which might ultimately result in a gain of weight. In fact, the chances are high that you might start feeling sluggish and bloated as you opt for overeating. Papaya comes filled with an enzyme known as papain. It helps by acting upon the proteins and also breaks them down. Having papaya in your daily diet can help in simplifying the process of digestion as you pair the same with food items that are rich in protein. Also, papaya acts as a great companion in the reduction of bloating.

Avocado

Some of you might have some doubts in mind after finding avocado in this listing of food items. Well, avocado is a super healthy food item, keeping aside the high calorific value it comes with. It comes filled with monosaturated fat, which helps a lot in keeping you satisfied and full for a long period of time. Including some slices of avocado with your daily meals can provide you enhanced strength to stay full for more time in case you opt for some difficult practice of fasting. Avocado also helps in dealing smartly with food cravings. So, if you are willing to stay away from the consumption of unhealthy snacks and food items, avocado is a great choice for you.

Potato

Potatoes can act as a superb companion for making all your meals a balanced one. They come with the capability of providing you with fast energy as they can be digested quite fast. There are people who try to stay away from consumption of potato as they think it is high in fat content. However, that is not the actual case. Potato can be coupled with other items, and avoid consuming them all alone. It can be included with all those food items that are rich in protein. You can also opt for potato as a quick snack after getting done with your schedule of workout. Our gut contains some good bacteria that help in the maintenance of a proper digestive system. Potatoes help in maintaining the health of the gut bacteria as well. In fact, consumption of potatoes can help you stay full for a longer time.

Fish

In accordance with the recent Dietary Guidelines, it is quite important to add at a minimum of eight ounces of fish to your overall diet per week. Well, it surely comes with some positive effects. Fish is a rich source of healthy fats and proteins as well. In fact, it comes with a great percentage of vitamin D too. As you begin with the regime of fasting, adding fish to your daily diet turns out to be even more essential. Having only one type of fish in your diet, you can easily provide your body with an entire dosage of all kinds of necessary nutrients. Also, fish acts as a great companion in improving the functioning of the brain.

Hummus

If you are a fan of dips and sauces, hummus is a great choice for you. In fact, it is considered the creamiest dips that are available today. It is also considered a superb source of protein that is derived from plants. You can include hummus in your daily diet for enhancing the nutrient content of various types of staples, such as sandwiches. If you want to opt for some snacks in between your fasting periods, you can prepare some tasty sandwiches along with some hummus for enhancing the taste. Add some meat-protein or veggies to the same for more nutrition. If you do not have enough time to prepare hummus on your own, you can opt for packaged hummus as well. If you want to prepare it on your own, just keep in mind that the secret ingredients for a rich hummus are tahini sauce and garlic.

__Cruciferous Vegetables__

Cruciferous veggies, such as broccoli, brussels sprouts, and cauliflower, are a great source of fiber. When you start with the program of intermittent fasting, adding enough fiber to your daily diet is quite necessary. Having all such vegetables can help you to deal with problems of constipation as they act as a great fiber source. In fact, you can also be sure of your bowel movements. Also, fiber is quite popular for providing satiety. So, you can opt for cruciferous veggies to stay full and satisfied for a long time. If you want to opt for fasting for twelve to sixteen hours, being full right before you start with the fast can help you achieve the best possible results.

Drinks

When you decide to start with intermittent fasting, opting for drinks and beverages can help you in staying hydrated for a longer time. You will also get the chance to control all your hunger pangs in a better way. There are certain drinks that you can have during your periods of fasting.

Water

No matter what kind of diet plan you opt for, you can never omit water from your life. Regardless of your eating pattern, you need to have enough water daily to keep your body properly hydrated. If you do not like to have normal water, you can opt for sparkling water to enhance the taste at the time of fasting. Adding a few drops of lemon juice to plain water is also a great option for enhancing the taste. However, try to stay away from adding any sort of sweetener. You can easily experiment with the water flavor by adding several ingredients, except for sugar. You can prepare a full jug of fruit-infused water by adding orange and cucumber slices to normal water. Doing so will help to make the fasting window a lot more interesting. If you try to add artificial sweeteners to water, it might readily interfere with the fasting results.

Coffee

Opting for a drink that comes with low or no calories is essential for the program of intermittent fasting. If you want to add some beverage to your daily diet, black coffee is a great option. You can also have normal coffee at the time of fasting. But you will have to make sure that you do not add any milk or any kind of sweetener to the coffee. Adding some spices for taste enhancement is allowed, such as cinnamon. One of the primary things that you will have to take care of while having coffee during your fasting period is the way you react to the same. There are people who tend to suffer from an upset stomach or racing heart after the consumption of coffee at the time of fasting. Having black coffee will help you in keeping the levels of blood sugar under control without the use of medication of any kind. In fact, it can also act as a superb energy booster during fasting as you might feel tired or lethargic when not provided with food for a long time.

Tea

Tea is a popular beverage that helps in enhancing satiety naturally. It can easily function as an effective tool to make the process of fasting a lot easier for you. Tea can also help in increasing your chances of succeeding with the program of intermittent fasting. You can select from the wide range of teas that are available in the market. It also acts as a popular beverage for enhancing the overall effectiveness of the program of intermittent fasting. Tea helps in supporting probiotic balance, improves gut health, along with cellular health. If you are trying to lose weight, nothing can be as useful as green tea.

Apple cider vinegar

Apple cider vinegar is a well-known product in today's world. It is mostly among all those people who are willing to lose weight. Consumption of apple cider vinegar helps in enhancing the effects of fasting. It can also provide needed help in proper maintenance of healthy levels of blood sugar, besides supporting proper digestion. In a recent study, it has been found that consumption of apple cider vinegar can help in improving the effects and results of intermittent fasting. If you do want to have apple cider vinegar alone, consider using the same as a dressing for your salads. Also, having apple cider vinegar with warm water helps in the proper movements of the bowel.

There are several other foods and drinks that you can include in your diet at the time of intermittent fasting. The options mentioned here are only a few of them. Just make sure you do not opt for any kind of food or drink that comes with high calorific value.

Chapter 7: Intermittent Fasting and Its Secrets

Intermittent fasting is a trending topic; however, there are certain secrets that are not known to most people. Having knowledge of all such secrets will surely help you in enhancing your weight loss goals besides other goals.

Tea: The Best Companion of Intermittent Fasting

We have already discussed how tea can be included in your intermittent fasting program. However, do you know that it comes with some other benefits as well besides aiding the program of intermittent fasting? Let us have a look at them.

- **Halts hunger:** The majority of people who opt for intermittent fasting tend to suffer from hunger pangs for the starting few weeks. That is primarily because of the fact that their body is used to have food for getting energy during the course of the day. Consumption of tea can help a lot in dealing with hunger pangs. Catechins present in tea tend to inhibit ghrelin secretion – the hormone which plays the part of signaling the body about hunger. So, you can easily be on track with your fasting program without any form of tension regarding your hunger pangs.

- **Enhances weight loss results:** Tea comes with no form of calories in it. So, consumption of the same helps in the enhancement of weight loss results. The catechins in tea also help in the promotion of fat loss. Additionally, the caffeine present in tea helps in increasing the energy expenditure besides fat oxidation. Thus, it helps in shedding excess pounds faster.

- **Helps in detox:** Consumption of tea while practicing intermittent fasting helps in initiating the natural detox process of the body called autophagy. The process gets triggered by the activation of certain proteins, which helps the body to throw out worn-out cells besides the regeneration of new cells.

For getting the best results, try to opt for about four cups of tea in one day to boost the overall effects of fasting. In order to experience the best impact, opt for cold brewing your tea. Cold-brewed tea comes with more antioxidants in comparison to normal steeped tea. It is because the hot water might burn a great portion of the antioxidants and catechins.

Water and Its Benefits

The most important benefit that comes along with the consumption of water at the time of fasting is detoxification. It is done by the process of autophagy, where the old and broken-down cells of the body are replenished. Water helps in enhancing the process of autophagy. Besides that, water also helps in lowering down blood pressure. Leptin and insulin are often considered the essential hormones that tend to affect the metabolism of the body. It has been found that consumption of water at the time of fasting enhances the effectiveness of these two hormones. Water also helps in lowering the risks of various chronic diseases. Dehydration can turn out to be one of the reasons for fatigue. No matter if you are only a bit dehydrated, it will surely affect your levels of cognition and concentration. Your body might also struggle to function in the proper way when the body is dehydrated. So, it can be said that water can act as a secret ingredient for enhancing the overall process of intermittent fasting.

Opt for Aromatherapy

If you are feeling low in energy while practicing intermittent fasting, you can opt for aromatherapy. Smell is often regarded as the strongest of all the senses. With proper usage of this sense, you can easily affect your brain functioning, productivity, and levels of energy in a positive way. Some of the scents that you can opt for are citrus, rosemary, peppermint, and lavender. You can opt for aromatherapy early in the morning to give your energy level a boost for the whole day's work.

Get Better Sleep

It is very natural to feel low in energy while being on a program of intermittent fasting. Well, to aid that, you will have to opt for a good night's sleep every day. Having a proper and sound sleep helps in boosting the levels of energy so that you can function the next day in the proper way, even without any kind of food. Try to create a bedtime routine and also stay away from alcohol consumption late in the day. Providing the body with enough rest is very important in intermittent fasting.

Chapter 8: Salad Recipes

Nothing can be as healthy as including salads in your diet plan, especially when you are trying to be on the program of intermittent fasting. Salads can provide you with more amount of nutrients, all in one place. You might think that including salads in your diet will make your overall diet plan quite dull. However, that is not the case. Salads can be prepared in several tasty ways that can provide you with nutrients and taste at the same time. You will find some superb and easy-to-make salad recipes in this section.

Walnut Cranberry Chicken Salad

Total Prep & Cooking Time: 15 minutes
Yields: Three servings
Nutrition Facts: Calories: 210.3 | Protein: 30.9g | Carbs: 10.7g | Fat: 14.2g | Fiber: 0.3g

Ingredients

- 15 ounces of chicken (canned in water)
- Half cup of Greek yogurt
- One tsp. of lemon juice
- ¼ cup of each

- Walnuts (chopped)
  - Cranberries (dried)
- Half tsp. of tarragon
- Six cups of chopped greens

Method:

1. Start by draining the water from the chicken with the help of a colander.
2. Transfer the drained chicken into a mixing bowl.
3. Add lemon juice, cranberries, walnuts, tarragon, and Greek yogurt.
4. Mix properly.
5. Serve the chicken salad with chopped green by the side.

Asparagus Balsamic Quinoa Salad and Baked Tofu

Total Prep & Cooking Time: 32 minutes
Yields: Six servings
Nutrition Facts: Calories: 224.6 | Protein: 8.7g | Carbs: 26.9g | Fat: 9.8g | Fiber: 5.1g

Ingredients

- One pound of asparagus (trimmed, cut into pieces of one inch)
- 1 ½ tbsps. of coconut oil
- One cup of quinoa (rinsed)
- 1 tbsp. of nutritional yeast
- Two cups of water
- Half tsp. of salad seasoning
- Six cups of baby spinach
- One avocado (pitted, sliced)
- Half cup of cucumber (chopped)

For the tofu:

- 13 ounces of tofu (dried, cut into small cubes)
- 3 tbsps. of balsamic vinegar

- 1 tsp. of maple syrup
- 2 tbsps. of soy sauce

Method:

1. Start by preparing the tofu.
2. Preheat your oven at 200 degrees Celsius.
3. Combine all the ingredients for the tofu in a baking dish.
4. Bake for twenty minutes.
5. In the meantime, prepare the asparagus.
6. Arrange the asparagus on a baking sheet.
7. Drizzle oil from the top.
8. Add pepper and salt.
9. Stir to coat.
10. Bake the asparagus for about ten minutes.
11. Prepare quinoa according to instructions on the package.
12. Add seasoning and yeast.
13. Create a base of spinach on a serving plate. Top with asparagus, quinoa, avocado, cucumber, and tofu.
14. Serve immediately.

Kale Salad

Total Prep & Cooking Time: 20 minutes
Yields: Three servings
Nutrition Facts: Calories: 140.8 | Protein: 5.6g | Carbs: 10.8g | Fat: 9.5g | Fiber: 4.8g

Ingredients

- One bunch of curly kale
- Half an avocado
- ¼ cup of red onion (sliced)
- Five ounces of cherry tomatoes
- 3 tbsps. of sunflower seeds

For the dressing:

- 2 tbsps. of tamari
- 3 tbsps. of lemon juice

Method:

1. Chop the kale into small pieces.
2. Transfer chopped kale to a bowl.
3. Massage lightly for tenderizing.

4. Add sliced onion to the bowl.
5. Add tamari along with lemon juice.
6. Toss properly for coating.
7. Dice avocado and tomato.
8. Add tomato and avocado to the salad.
9. Toss again.
10. Combine the dressing ingredients in a bowl.
11. Drizzle the dressing over the salad.
12. Toss the salad to coat.
13. Top with sunflower seeds before serving.

Chicken Salad

Total Prep & Cooking Time: 15 minutes
Yields: Three servings
Nutrition Facts: Calories: 230.7 | Protein: 27.8g | Carbs: 10.1g | Fat: 16.5g | Fiber: 2.1g

Ingredients

- one cup of Greek yogurt (plain)
- Half tsp. of garlic powder
- ¼ tsp. of each
    - Black pepper (ground)
    - Salt
- Two cups of chicken (cooked, diced)
- 2 tbsps. of red onion (diced)
- Half cup of apple (diced)
- 1/3 cup of green celery (diced)
- ¼ cup of almonds (sliced)

Method:

1. Start by combining garlic powder, salt, pepper, and Greek yogurt in a bowl.

2. Combine the remaining ingredients with the yogurt mixture in a large bowl.

3. Serve with bread or as a salad.

Arugula Strawberry Salad With Balsamic Vinaigrette

Total Prep & Cooking Time: 10 minutes
Yields: Three servings
Nutrition Facts: Calories: 220.8 | Protein: 17.9g | Carbs: 12.4g | Fat: 22.7g | Fiber: 3.2g

Ingredients

- Six cups of arugula
- Six ounces of each
    - Blueberries
    - Raspberries
- One cup of strawberries
- ¼ cup of almonds (slivered)
- Half cup of feta cheese

For the vinaigrette:

- ¼ cup of each
    - Olive oil
    - Balsamic vinegar
- Three teaspoons of sugar

- Half tsp. of Dijon mustard
- Pepper and salt

Method:

1. Combine all the listed ingredients for the salad in a bowl.
2. Stir together the vinaigrette ingredients in a small bowl.
3. Pour the vinaigrette all over the salad.
4. Toss well to coat.
5. Divide the salad into serving bowls and serve.

Shrimp Caesar Salad

Total Prep & Cooking Time: 20 minutes
Yields: Four servings
Nutrition Facts: Calories: 210.8 | Protein: 22.8g | Carbs: 17.9g | Fat: 5.5g | Fiber: 1.9g

Ingredients

For the salad:

- Two cups of garlic croutons
- Eight cups of lettuce (romaine, chopped)
- ¼ cup of parmesan cheese (shredded)

For the shrimp:

- One pound of shrimp (peeled, deveined)
- 1 tsp. of olive oil
- Pepper and salt
- 2 tbsps. of lemon juice

For the dressing:

- Half cup of yogurt (plain)
- 1 ½ tbsps. of Dijon mustard
- One clove of garlic

- 2 tbsps. of each
    - Lemon juice
    - Parmesan cheese (grated)
- Pepper and salt
- 3 tbsps. of water

Method:

1. Start by combining croutons and lettuce in a bowl.
2. Combine olive oil, shrimp, pepper, and salt in another bowl.
3. Grill the shrimps in a grill pan for about three minutes.
4. Transfer grilled shrimps to a bowl.
5. Toss with lemon juice.
6. Combine all the listed ingredients for the salad dressing in a food processor.
7. Add dressing and shrimps to the lettuce mixture.
8. Toss well to combine.
9. Garnish with cheese and serve.

Broccoli Salad

Total Prep & Cooking Time: 10 minutes
Yields: Six servings
Nutrition Facts: Calories: 256.9 | Protein: 8.1g | Carbs: 22.4g | Fat: 16.8g | Fiber: 4.2g

Ingredients

- One cup of mayonnaise
- 2 tbsps. of red wine vinegar
- 1/3 cup of sugar
- 1 tsp. of celery seed
- 12 ounces of bacon (cooked, chopped)
- Two broccoli heads (broken into florets)
- Half cup of almond (slivered, toasted)
- ¾ cup of celery (chopped)
- Two green onions (sliced thinly)
- 2 cups of seedless grapes (red, halved)

Method:

1. Combine sugar, mayonnaise, celery seed, and vinegar in a bowl.

2. Let the mixture sit in the refrigerator for half an hour.

3. Mix together bacon, broccoli, green onion, almonds, grapes, and celery in a bowl.

4. Pour the dressing from the top.

5. Toss well to coat.

6. Divide the salad among serving bowls and serve.

Roasted Beet and Blood Orange Salad

Total Prep & Cooking Time: One hour
Yields: Four servings
Nutrition Facts: Calories: 167.8 | Protein: 4.5g | Carbs: 22.8g | Fat: 2.7g | Fiber: 5.3g

Ingredients

- One pound of beet (scrubbed clean)
- Pepper and salt
- Four cups of each
    - Butter lettuce (torn)
    - Baby spinach
    - Blood orange (peeled, chopped)
- ¼ cup of feta cheese
- One avocado (diced)

For the dressing:

- Half tsp. of thyme
- ¼ cup of walnuts (toasted)
- 2 tbsps. of lemon juice

- One clove of garlic (minced)
- 1/3 cup of olive oil

Method:

1. Preheat your oven to 210 degrees Celsius.
2. Rub beets with oil.
3. Sprinkle with pepper and salt.
4. Wrap the seasoned beets in aluminum foil.
5. Roast in the oven for forty minutes.
6. Cube the roasted beets.
7. Combine the remaining ingredients along with the roasted beets in a bowl.
8. Combine the dressing ingredients in a small bowl.
9. Drizzle the dressing over the salad.
10. Toss well to coat.
11. Serve immediately.

Spinach Salad

Total Prep & Cooking Time: 10 minutes
Yields: Three servings
Nutrition Facts: Calories: 42.8 | Protein: 3.7g | Carbs: 5.6g | Fat: 2.9g | Fiber: 2.2g

Ingredients

- Eight ounces of spinach
- Four cups of water
- One green onion (chopped)
- One garlic clove (minced)
- Two teaspoons of each
    - Sesame oil
    - Soy sauce
- ½ tsp. of sesame seeds (toasted)
- Pepper and salt

Method:

1. Wash the spinach under cold running water.
2. Cut off the spinach roots.

3. Blanch the spinach in boiling water for thirty seconds.

4. Rinse the spinach using cold water.

5. Squeeze out any excess water.

6. Combine green onion, garlic, sesame oil, soy sauce, sesame seeds, and spinach in a bowl.

7. Add pepper and salt.

8. Toss to combine.

9. Serve immediately.

Buckwheat Salad

Total Prep & Cooking Time: 15 minutes
Yields: Five servings
Nutrition Facts: Calories: 302.8 | Protein: 17.9g | Carbs: 33.6g | Fat: 7.9g | Fiber: 3.7g

Ingredients

- Four cups of mixed greens
- Half cup of white buckwheat (raw)
- Two tomatoes (chopped)
- One onion (chopped)
- 1/3 cup of each
    - Cranberries (dried)
    - Pumpkin seeds
    - Rice wine vinegar
- Three teaspoons of sesame oil
- Pepper and salt

Method:

1. To cook the buckwheat, mix buckwheat groats with two cups of water.

2. Boil the mixture.

3. Cook for ten minutes.

4. Combine cooked buckwheat with remaining salad ingredients in a bowl.

5. Divide the salad among serving bowls and serve.

Chapter 9: Meat Recipes

Meat forms an essential part of any kind of diet, and the same goes for intermittent fasting as well. Including meat in your diet plan will provide you with a great dose of protein along with various other essential nutrients that can help you to stay energized and functional during the course of fasting.

<u>Mediterranean-Style Chicken Breast and Avocado Tapenade</u>

Total Prep & Cooking Time: 45 minutes
Yields: Three servings
Nutrition Facts: Calories: 270.8 | Protein: 24.9g | Carbs: 7.2g | Fat: 14.6g | Fiber: 3.4g

Ingredients

- Three chicken breast halves (skinless)
- 5 tbsps. of lemon juice
- 1 tbsp. of lemon peel (grated)
- Two tbsps. of olive oil
- One clove of garlic (chopped)
- Half tsp. of salt
- ¼ tsp. of black pepper (ground)
- Two cloves of garlic (roasted, mashed)

- One tomato (chopped)
- ¼ cup of green pimento-stuffed olive (sliced)
- 3 tbsps. of capers (rinsed)
- 2 tbsps. of basil (sliced)
- One avocado (chopped)

Method:

1. Combine chicken, lemon peel, two tablespoons of lemon juice, olive oil, salt, pepper, and garlic in a sealable plastic bag.
2. Place in the refrigerator for twenty minutes.
3. Combine remaining lemon juice, olive oil, pepper, salt, and roasted garlic in a bowl.
4. Add green olives, tomato, capers, avocado, and basil.
5. Mix well.
6. Discard the marinade.
7. Grill the chicken in a pan for five minutes on each side.
8. Serve the grilled chicken hot with avocado tapenade by the side.

__Veggie Cheesy Chicken Salad Sandwich__

Total Prep & Cooking Time: 25 minutes
Yields: Two servings
Nutrition Facts: Calories: 322.8 | Protein: 51.9g | Carbs: 10.8g | Fat: 9.2g | Fiber: 3.1g

Ingredients

- One cup of chicken breast (cooked, cubed)
- ¼ cup of each
    - Celery (chopped)
    - Carrot (shaved in ribbons)
    - Cheddar cheese (shredded)
- Half cup of baby spinach (chopped)
- 3 tbsps. of mayonnaise
- 2 tbsps. of sour cream
- 1/8 tsp. of parslcy (dried)
- 2 ½ tbsps. of Dijon mustard
- Four slices of bread

Method:

1. Combine all the ingredients except for the bread slices in a bowl.

2. Chill the salad mixture in the refrigerator for half an hour.

3. Divide the chicken mixture among bread slices.

4. Serve immediately.

Brussel Sprouts and Chicken

Total Prep & Cooking Time: 55 minutes
Yields: Four servings
Nutrition Facts: Calories: 312.8 | Protein: 17.2g | Carbs: 6.8g | Fat: 22.9g | Fiber: 2.8g

Ingredients

- Four chicken thighs
- Two cups of brussels sprouts (halved)
- Four large carrots (bias cut)
- One tsp. of herb mixture
- 3 tbsps. of olive oil

Method:

1. Combine all the veggies in a bowl.
2. Add pepper, salt, half teaspoon of the herb mixture, and two tablespoons of olive oil.
3. Toss to combine.
4. Arrange the vegetables on a sheet pan.
5. Marinade the chicken thighs with the remaining ingredients.
6. Place the chicken thighs on the pan.
7. Roast for thirty minutes in the oven.
8. Serve warm.

Easy Beef Steak With Hollandaise Sauce and Grilled Asparagus

Total Prep & Cooking Time: 50 minutes
Yields: Two servings
Nutrition Facts: Calories: 656.8 | Protein: 67.8g | Carbs: 6.7g | Fat: 70.8g | Fiber: 3.9g

Ingredients

For the steak:

- Two beef sirloin steaks
- One tsp. of olive oil
- Pepper and salt

For the sauce:

- One stick of butter
- Three egg yolks
- 2 tbsps. of sun-dried tomatoes (chopped)
- Two teaspoons of lemon juice
- 1 tbsp. of basil (chopped)
- Pepper and salt

For the asparagus:

- Sixteen spears of asparagus (trimmed, halved)
- 1 tbsp. of olive oil
- Pepper and salt

Method:

1. Melt the butter in the microwave.
2. Add the remaining listed ingredients for the sauce in a jar along with the butter.
3. Use a hand blender and blend the ingredients.
4. Toss the asparagus with olive oil, pepper, and salt.
5. Grill the asparagus for ten minutes.
6. Rub the steaks with olive oil, pepper, and salt.
7. Cook the steaks on the grill for five minutes on each side.
8. Serve the steaks warm with grilled asparagus and drizzle hollandaise sauce from the top.

Chimichurri Chicken Tray Bake

Total Prep & Cooking Time: 48 minutes
Yields: Four servings
Nutrition Facts: Calories: 626.8 | Protein: 22.8g | Carbs: 7.8g | Fat: 52.7g | Fiber: 4.6g

Ingredients

- Four chicken thighs (with skin and bone)
- One tsp. of onion powder
- Pepper and salt
- Half tsp. of garlic powder
- Five ounces of each
    - Green beans
    - Asparagus
    - Sliced florets of broccoli

For the chimichurri:

- One cup of parsley
- ¼ cup of oregano
- Six cloves of garlic
- Half cup of olive oil
- Four tbsps. of red wine vinegar

- Pepper and salt

Method:

1. Preheat the microwave to 200 degrees Celsius.
2. Combine all the dry seasonings together in a bowl.
3. Rub the seasoning on the chicken thighs.
4. Arrange the chicken on a baking tray with the skin side up.
5. Cook for about twenty minutes.
6. Remove the tray from the oven.
7. Scatter the greens all over the chicken.
8. Cover the tray with aluminum foil.
9. Cook for fifteen minutes.
10. Add all the chimichurri ingredients to a food processor.
11. Blend until smooth.
12. Serve the veggies and chicken warm with a drizzle of chimichurri from the top.

Capsicum and Cheese Stuffed Meatloaf

Total Prep & Cooking Time: One hour and thirty minutes
Yields: Two servings
Nutrition Facts: Calories: 467.8 | Protein: 28.8g | Carbs: 5.3g | Fat: 32.6g | Fiber: 3.5g

Ingredients

- One pound of beef (minced)
- One yellow onion (chopped)
- Two large eggs
- Two teaspoons of garlic (minced)
- 1/3 cup of flax meal
- 2 tbsps. of coconut aminos
- 4 tbsps. of tomato passata
- 1 tbsp. of fresh herbs (minced)
- One capsicum (chopped)
- Half cup of cheddar cheese (shredded)
- Seven ounces of Gouda cheese
- ¼ cup of parmesan cheese (grated)

For baste:

- 4 tbsps. of tomato passata
- 2 tbsps. of coconut aminos

Method:

1. Preheat the microwave to 180 degrees Celsius.
2. Add beef, eggs, garlic, onion, flax meal, passata, coconut aminos, and herbs in a bowl.
3. Use your hands and combine them properly.
4. Use silicone paper for lining a baking tray.
5. Lay a silicone paper on a working surface.
6. Add the beef mixture on top of the paper.
7. Give the meat mixture the shape of a flat rectangle using your fingers.
8. Arrange the gouda slices over the meatloaf.
9. You can overlap the slices if needed.

10. Sprinkle capsicum all over the capsicum, along with cheddar and parmesan cheese.

11. Start rolling the meat mixture as tightly as possible.

12. Carefully peel the silicone paper back as you keep rolling.

13. Pinch the meatloaf ends so that cheese does not ooze out.

14. Place the rolled meatloaf on the prepared baking tray.

15. Cover the tray with aluminum foil.

16. Bake the meatloaf for fifteen minutes.

17. Remove the foil.

18. Bale again for fifteen minutes.

19. Mix the ingredients for the baste in a bowl.

20. Baste the meatloaf as much as you want to.

21. Cut the meatloaf into slices.

22. Serve warm.

Steak Taco Bowl

Total Prep & Cooking Time: 20 minutes
Yields: One serving
Nutrition Facts: Calories: 513.8 | Protein: 28.5g | Carbs: 7.3g | Fat: 55.4g | Fiber: 7.6g

Ingredients

- One small steak
- One tbsp. of butter
- Pepper and salt
- One cup of cauliflower rice (cooked)
- 2 tbsps. of cilantro (minced)
- One teaspoon of lime juice

For the toppings:

- Half an avocado (sliced)
- ¼ cup of tomato salsa
- One tbsp. of sour cream
- Half a jalapeno pepper (sliced)
- Two radishes (sliced thinly)

Method:

1. Start by heating butter in a small iron skillet.
2. Use pepper and salt for seasoning the steak.
3. Add the steak to the skillet.
4. Sear for six minutes on each side.
5. Let the steak rest for five minutes on a cutting board.
6. Combine cauliflower rice with lime juice and cilantro in a bowl.
7. Top the rice with the toppings.
8. Slice the steak and add the slices over the rice.
9. Serve immediately.

Caprese Chicken Bowl

Total Prep & Cooking Time: 45 minutes
Yields: One serving
Nutrition Facts: Calories: 578.6 | Protein: 41.8g | Carbs: 5.7g | Fat: 53.8g | Fiber: 8.9g

Ingredients

For the chicken:

- One chicken breast (skinless, boneless)
- 1 tbsp. of olive oil
- One teaspoon of balsamic vinegar
- Pepper and salt
- Half tsp. of Italian seasoning

For the salad:

- Two cups of spinach
- ¼ cup of basil leaves
- Two ounces of mozzarella cheese (sliced)
- Half an avocado (sliced)
- 1/3 cup of cherry tomatoes (halved)

For the dressing:

- One tbsp. of olive oil
- One teaspoon of balsamic vinegar
- Pepper and salt

Method:

1. Place the chicken breast with Italian seasoning, olive oil, pepper, and salt in a sealable plastic bag.
2. Keep in the refrigerator for ten minutes.
3. Heat an iron skillet over a medium flame.
4. Sear the chicken breast for five minutes on each side.
5. Slice the chicken breast.
6. Combine all the ingredients for the dressing in a bowl.
7. Arrange the salad by placing mozzarella and vegetables in a bowl.
8. Top the salad with sliced chicken.
9. Drizzle the dressing all over the salad and chicken.
10. Serve immediately.

Chapter 10: Seafood Recipes

Besides providing you with great taste, seafood comes with great quantities of omega-3 fatty acids. You can include seafood in your daily meal plan for enjoying the rich taste and goodness of nutrients as well. You will find some easy-to-make seafood recipes in this chapter that you can have while practicing intermittent fasting.

Cod Loin With Browned Butter and Horseradish

Total Prep & Cooking Time: 35 minutes
Yields: Four servings
Nutrition Facts: Calories: 410.6 | Protein: 32.1g | Carbs: 6.5g | Fat: 28.7g | Fiber: 4.2g

Ingredients

- Two pounds of cod (no bone fillet)
- One teaspoon of salt
- 3 ounces of horseradish (grated)
- Five ounces of butter
- One pound of green beans
- Pepper and salt
- One ounce of celery root (sliced)

Method:

1. Season the fillets of cod using salt.
2. Keep in the refrigerator for half an hour.
3. Use paper towels for drying the fish fillets.
4. Heat about one-third of the butter in an iron skillet.
5. Fry the fish fillets for four minutes on each side.
6. Keep basting the fish fillets with the pan butter so that the fillets do not dry out.
7. Season with pepper.
8. Remove the fish fillets from the skillet and place them on a cutting board.
9. Melt the remaining butter in a small saucepan until it gets light brown in color.
10. Boil the green beans in salted water for two minutes.
11. Place the fish fillet on a bed of cooked beans.
12. Drizzle browned butter from the top.
13. Top with grated horseradish.
14. Serve warm.

**Creamy Fish Casserole**

Total Prep & Cooking Time: 45 minutes
Yields: Four servings
Nutrition Facts: Calories: 626.8 | Protein: 36.8g | Carbs: 7.7g | Fat: 61.8g | Fiber: 4.5g

Ingredients

- One tbsp. of butter
- 3 tbsps. of olive oil
- One pound of broccoli (cut in small florets)
- One tsp. of salt
- Half tsp. of black pepper (ground)
- Four ounces of scallions (chopped)
- 2 tbsps. of small capers
- Two pounds of white fish (cut in small pieces)
- 1 ½ tbsps. of parsley (dried)
- Two cups of whipping cream
- 1 1/3 tbsps. of Dijon mustard
- Three ounces of butter (cut in equal slices)

Method:

1. Preheat the microwave oven to 200 degrees Celsius.
2. Use butter for greasing a baking dish.
3. Heat oil in a large pan.
4. Add the florets of broccoli.
5. Stir-fry the florets for five minutes.
6. Add pepper and salt.
7. Add capers and scallions to the pan.
8. Cook for two minutes.
9. Transfer the broccoli mixture into the greased baking dish.
10. Arrange the fish on top of the veggies.
11. Whisk together whipping cream, parsley, and mustard in a bowl.
12. Pour the mixture over the veggies and fish.
13. Top with pieces of sliced butter.
14. Bake the fish and veggies for twenty minutes.
15. Serve warm.

Sesame Crusted Salmon and Cauli-Rice

Total Prep & Cooking Time: 25 minutes
Yields: Two servings
Nutrition Facts: Calories: 624.8 | Protein: 44.9g | Carbs: 7.6g | Fat: 60.5g | Fiber: 6.1g

Ingredients

For the fish:

- Two fillets of wild salmon
- ¼ cup of sesame seeds
- 2 tbsps. of coconut oil

For the cauliflower rice:

- Half a cauliflower
- 2 tbsps. of coconut oil
- 1 tsp. of erythritol
- Half tsp. of salt
- 1/3 cup of coconut cream
- ¼ cup of cilantro

Method:

1. Start by placing cauliflower in a blender by cutting the cauliflower into small florets.

2. Keep blending until it resembles rice.

3. Heat coconut oil in a large pan.

4. Add the processed cauliflower.

5. Cook for five minutes.

6. Add salt and erythritol.

7. Add the coconut cream and mix well.

8. Add the cilantro.

9. Keep aside.

10. Heat another medium pan over medium heat.

11. Place the sesame seeds in a shallow dish.

12. Coat the fish fillets in sesame seeds on all sides.

13. Add coconut oil to the pan.

14. Add the fillets of salmon.

15. Cook for eight minutes on each side.

16. Divide the cooked cauliflower rice among serving plates.

17. Top with cooked salmon fillet.

18. Garnish with cilantro.

19. Serve warm.

Crab Zucchini Melts

Total Prep & Cooking Time: 45 minutes
Yields: Four servings
Nutrition Facts: Calories: 598.5 | Protein: 28.7g | Carbs: 6.2g | Fat: 55.7g | Fiber: 3.3g

Ingredients

- Two zucchinis
- One tbsp. of olive oil
- Three ounces of celery stalks
- 12 ounces of crab meat
- One red bell pepper
- ¾ cup of mayonnaise
- 1 ½ tbsps. of Dijon mustard
- Seven ounces of cheddar cheese (shredded)
- Pepper and salt

For serving:

- 2 tbsps. of olive oil
- Four ounces of baby spinach
- Pepper and salt

Method:

1. Start by preheating the microwave to 225 degrees Celsius.
2. Slice the zucchinis lengthwise.
3. Use a spoon for scooping out a trench right in the middle for the filling.
4. Use a paper towel for pat drying the zucchinis.
5. Chop celery and bell pepper finely.
6. Use parchment paper for lining a baking sheet.
7. Brush the zucchinis with olive oil.
8. Arrange the zucchinis on the baking sheet.
9. Bake for seven minutes.
10. Combine chopped veggies with mayonnaise, crab meat, Dijon mustard, and cheese.
11. Add pepper and salt.
12. Spoon the crab mixture onto the baked zucchini slices.
13. Bake for twenty minutes.
14. Serve the crab zucchini melts with baby spinach and a light drizzle of olive oil.

Seared Salmon With Lemony Sauce

Total Prep & Cooking Time: 40 minutes
Yields: Two servings
Nutrition Facts: Calories: 689.5 | Protein: 54.3g | Carbs: 6.8g | Fat: 73.6g | Fiber: 5.3g

Ingredients

- Half cup of vegetable stock
- 2/3 cup of whipping cream
- One tbsp. of chives (chopped)
- 2 tbsps. of parsley (chopped)
- Half a lemon (juiced)
- Half tsp. of salt
- One pinch of black pepper (ground)
- 2 ½ tbsps. of olive oil
- One pound of salmon
- Pepper and salt

For serving:

- One tbsp. of butter
- Fifteen cups of spinach

- Pepper and salt

Method:

1. Add the vegetable stock into a saucepan.
2. Boil the vegetable stock for a few minutes.
3. Add chives, cream, lemon juice, parsley, pepper, and salt.
4. Whisk well to combine.
5. Reduce the flame and keep whisking.
6. Let the sauce thicken.
7. Heat olive oil in an iron skillet.
8. Season the fish with pepper and salt on all sides.
9. Add the salmon to the skillet with the skin side down.
10. Sear for four minutes on each side.
11. Melt the butter in a wok.
12. Add the spinach.
13. Toss the spinach for a couple of minutes until wilted.
14. Add pepper and salt.
15. Serve salmon by drizzling lemon sauce from the top and spinach by the side.

**Smoked Mussels Casserole**

Total Prep & Cooking Time: 30 minutes
Yields: Four servings
Nutrition Facts: Calories: 660.3 | Protein: 28.7g | Carbs: 8.7g | Fat: 73.8g | Fiber: 4.7g

Ingredients

- One pound of cauliflower
- 2 tbsps. of Dijon mustard
- 2 ounces of onion (chopped)
- One cup of mayonnaise
- Seven ounces of cheddar cheese (shredded)
- 2 ½ tbsps. of chives
- 10 ounces of smoked mussels (canned)
- Pepper and salt

For serving:

- Four tbsps. of olive oil
- Eight ounces of leafy greens

Method:

1. Preheat the microwave to 200 degrees Celsius.
2. Cut the cauliflower into florets.
3. Place the florets in a pot.
4. Cover the florets with water.
5. Add salt to the pot.
6. Boil for five minutes.
7. Drain the water.
8. Combine mustard, onion, two-third of the cheese, and mayonnaise in a bowl.
9. Add mussels and cauliflower to the mixture.
10. Blend the mixture.
11. Pour the mixture into a baking dish.
12. Sprinkle with remaining cheese from the top.
13. Bake for about fifteen minutes.
14. Serve warm with olive oil and leafy greens.

Harissa Shrimp Skewers

Total Prep & Cooking Time: One hour and twenty minutes
Yields: Four servings
Nutrition Facts: Calories: 165.3 | Protein: 15.6g | Carbs: 2.7g | Fat: 8.5g | Fiber: 0.2g

Ingredients

- One pound of shrimp (large, peeled, deveined)
- Pepper and salt
- 3 tbsps. of butter (melted)
- 1 tbsp. of lime juice
- 2 tbsps. of harissa paste
- Two cloves of garlic (minced)
- One lime (cut in wedges, to serve)
- Four skewers

Method:

1. Start by seasoning the shrimps using pepper and salt.

2. Add harissa, butter, lime juice, garlic, and salt in a bowl.

3. Combine properly.

4. Add the seasoned shrimps to the bowl.

5. Toss for coating in the sauce.

6. Let the shrimp rest for about one hour.

7. Thread the marinated shrimps into the skewers.

8. Pour the leftover marinade all over the shrimp.

9. Heat a grill pan over a medium flame.

10. Add the skewers.

11. Roast the shrimps for five minutes, turning occasionally.

12. Serve warm with lime wedges

Chapter 11: Activities to Opt For

Living with extra pounds might turn out to be quite uncomfortable, especially if you are suffering from obesity for a long time. In fact, an excess amount of fat in the body can trigger chronic health problems. Well, the cases related to obesity have reached new heights in the last few years, probably because of the kind of lifestyle that people tend to lead to today. Some of the most widely found problems that get triggered by obesity are diabetes, chronic heart problems, stroke, and many others. When it comes to weight loss, intermittent fasting can provide you with the desired outcome in no time at all. You will also have to opt for certain activities like yoga and exercises to enhance the overall results.

Physical Activities to Enhance the Effectivity of Intermittent Fasting

Working out while being in a fasted state can readily help you to lose weight within a short period of time. But if you are opting for fasting for long time periods, such as 24 hours or 48 hours, then it is always suggested to opt for low-intensity workouts.

- **Walking:** Walking is always considered a low-intensity exercise and is something that can be easily managed while being on an empty stomach. Waling for about half an hour every day while being in the fasted state can help in the burning of calories and ultimately results in weight loss.

- **Yoga:** It cannot be said that yoga directly helps in losing weight; however, while being on a program of intermittent fasting, it is quite essential to be relaxed and focused. Yoga can provide you with the needed help to stay calm and relaxed. It can also help in diverting your mind every time when you feel hungry during the window of fasting. On all those days when you are feeling quite low in energy or when you are trying to adjust your lifestyle with intermittent fasting, yoga will be easier for your body.

- **Strength training:** To properly build muscle mass, it is essential to fuel the body with all forms of carbs and proteins, either before or after working out. If you are willing to increase your mass, then it is always suggested to train yourself either before breaking your fast or during the eating window. It is not recommended to opt for exercising at the end of the eating window as you won't be able to recover that much. You will have to balance your workout goals with the food that you eat. If you feel depleted while working out, then something might not be right. Try to tweak the food items that you include in your diet to fill that gap.

- **Cardio:** When carried out in the perfect way, fasted cardio can provide you with great results. If you are trying to opt for a slow morning run, you can easily wait for some hours after running to have your meals. However, if you feel dizzy and weak, try to have a meal after getting done with your cardio. Slowly moving forward with low-intensity workouts will help you to adjust yourself to an extensive workout routine in the later phase.

There are various other exercise options that you can opt for while being in the fasted state. We will discuss the same in the later chapters.

Benefits of Exercising While Practicing Intermittent Fasting

Right before you start with intermittent fasting with the aim of losing excess pounds or for some possible reasons, you might have a question in your mind – "Can I continue with my workout schedule?" Well, yes can keep following your schedule of workout. However, there are certain benefits and downsides as well that you will have to pay attention to. Exercising while being in a fasted state can affect muscle biochemistry to a great extent, besides the metabolic rate. There is also some research that suggests consumption of food and then working out immediately, much before digestion starts. When you decide to exercise in the fasted state, the stored body carbohydrates termed glycogen start getting depleted at a faster rate. As a result, it will lead to more burning down of fat to provide fuel to your routine of exercise.

However, before you make up your mind to get started with fasted cardio, there is a downside as well. When you opt for exercising at the time of fasting, the body might start breaking down your muscles to use up the protein as energy. That is why a heavy workout is not suggested while being on intermittent fasting. The main reason behind this is that the body might deplete itself with calories and energy. Also, there is evidence that suggests exercising in the fasted state helps in speeding up the process of fat burning. It can be said that whether exercising or other physical activities at the time of intermittent fasting will suit you or not will depend on your physical condition. For some, it works great, and for others, it does not. So, before you start with any kind of activity, try to consult a doctor.

Extent of Exercises for Weight Loss While Practicing Intermittent Fasting

In order to enjoy all the possible benefits of working out, it is always suggested to get indulged in several types of aerobic exercises for at least twenty minutes. Give your best to be on this schedule about three times every week. You can extend the session beyond twenty minutes; however, as you will be in the fasted state, it is not suggested to opt for extensive periods of exercise. You can also opt for moderate exercises if you do not feel that energized to opt for heavy exercises. You can start with walking or jogging every day for about fifteen minutes. If you are able to burn out about 600 calories every week, you will be able to lose about ten pounds of weight during the course of the year.

How to Get Started With a Proper Workout Session While Fasting?

If you have decided to continue your schedule of workout at the time of fasting, there are certain important points that you will have to keep in mind.

Paying attention to timing

In order to get the best results from exercising, you will have to pay attention to three considerations – whether to exercise before, after, or during the eating window. The most common type of intermittent fasting is the 16/8 method. As we already know, you will have to maintain your fast for 16 hours straight with an eating window of 8 hours. Opting for physical activities before the eating window might turn out to be the most effective for all those people who can give their best while being on an empty stomach. Exercising during the eating window will be the best option if you cannot exercise on an empty stomach. It is often suggested to opt for physical activities during the eating window for fast recovery and best performance. Working out after the eating window will be a good option for all those who like to exercise after getting their level of energy at the peak.

The time that you select for working out needs to be decided after paying attention to the responses of the body. If you are not sure which time slot will suit you the best, you can test all of them to find the perfect one.

Having proper meals

The perfect way of pairing up intermittent fasting with exercising is by placing the exercise timing right during the eating window. It is because, during the eating window, your nutrition level will reach its peak. In case you opt for heavy lifting, it is important for the body to get enough proteins after getting done with the exercise session in order to aid regeneration. You can try to consume carbs after weight training besides 20 grams of proteins within thirty minutes of getting done with your exercise.

Deciding the type of exercise based on macros

It is quite an important thing to pay attention to the macronutrients that you consume every day right before working out and also while you have your food afterward. For example, weight training needs more carbs, whereas high-intensity exercises and cardio can be carried out with lower carbs.

Working Out Safely At the Time of Fasting

The rate of success of any exercise program or weight loss program depends completely on the limit of its safety and also whether it can be sustained in the long term. If your target is to reduce the body fat percentage and also maintain the proper level of fitness while doing intermittent fasting, it is important to be in the safe zone. Here are some tips that might help you to stay safe.

- **Taking care of the electrolytes:** You need to maintain the level of the electrolyte all the time at the time of working out. You can opt for coconut water for replenishing the electrolytes. It comes with a low-calorie count and also tastes good. If you are thinking of opting for flavored energy drinks, it will be better for you if you can stay away from them. It is because flavored energy drinks come with high sugar content.

- **Having meals close to your exercise session:** The timing of your meals always plays an essential role in your exercise sessions. The key to reaping all the benefits of working out is to place your meals in close proximity to your sessions of workout. Doing so will help the body to use up all the stored glycogen in order to provide fuel for exercise. You can also opt for some protein supplements after getting done with your exercise to build more lean muscles.

- **Staying hydrated:** Being on a program intermittent fasting does not indicate that you will have to stay away from water. Exercising while fasting needs a great amount of water. It helps in keeping the body hydrated all the time.

- **Taking care of the duration and intensity:** If you try to push your body hard from the very beginning, it might readily result in dizziness and fatigue. The moment you feel that you can no longer take the load, try taking a break. Properly listening to the body in all such situations is the best way in which complexities can be avoided. There is no need to force your body. In case you are stressing a lot on your body at the time of working out, reduce the intensity of your workout session along with the duration for the first two to three weeks.

Chapter 12: Five Commonly Made Mistakes

Your friend was able to lose about 15 pounds, and you are not even able to stop yourself from being sure of the weight-loss merits of intermittent fasting. There are people who just think of intermittent fasting as some sort of fancy name that comes with the only aim of skipping your breakfast. However, that is not true. Having such thoughts in mind will surely lead you in the direction of making mistakes. As you make such mistakes, you might not be able to see the actual benefits of the diet. What could be worse if you just end up making yourself dehydrated or miserable. Maybe you have developed a routine that just feels good to you; however, for some reason, the benefits cannot be seen. You might be on a regime that is helping you to shed weight; however, it is leaving you exhausted and in a devastating state for the rest of the day. In actuality, intermittent fasting won't work the same for everyone.

There are certain mistakes that most beginners tend to make and all it results in is a complete failure.

Jumping Into Intermittent Fasting Too Fast

Well, there are levels to everything. One of the primary reasons why a majority of the diets do not show any kind of benefit is the extreme gap from the usual – the natural way of eating. As you try to depart to a great extent from the actual, it will naturally feel impossible for you to maintain the same. If you are just starting with intermittent fasting and you have the habit of consuming food after every two hours or so, try not to opt for a hardcore fast, like fasting for 24 hours straight, from the beginning. You will have to opt for an adjustment period that needs to be natural and should also feel good at the same time. The human body is surprisingly a superb communicator. It will always signal you whether something feels like not the 'right fit.' There is nothing to say that fasting yourself for 24 hours will surely make you feel irritated and tired.

If you are sure of the concept of fasting, try to start with 12 hours fast. Opt for fasting for 12 hours every day and consume food during the other half of the day. That would be quite close to what you are actually used to doing, and it might also turn out to be the most sustainable plan to follow for the long term. Once the plan starts feeling comfortable to you, you can move one level up to the 16:8 method of intermittent fasting, where you will have an eating window of eight hours during the course of the day. What makes intermittent fasting so popular is its flexibility. So, try to opt for a plan that will help you to be fixated on a time period without making you feel terrible.

Choosing the Wrong Plan

Try not to set yourself up for disappointment by opting for something that you are aware of might cramp your lifestyle. Maintaining a number of miserable fasting days right before you opt for a 24-hour food party won't help you with anything. Intermittent fasting is all about making certain changes that can be maintained. For instance, if you have the habit of staying awake all night, it will be better for you if you do not start fasting early in the morning. If you are a heavy workout enthusiast and you are not ready to sacrifice your daily gym routine, try not to opt for a plan that will restrict your calories for few days every week. No one else will know your lifestyle better than you. So, you are the expert here, and you will have to opt for the plan wisely that will fit seamlessly with your lifestyle.

Consuming Excessive Food During the Eating Window

It can be regarded as the most common trap that the majority of people practicing intermittent fasting tend to fall into. If you have opted for a restrictive plan that keeps you hungry for a long time or for the majority of the day, the chances are high that you might just get indulged in overeating every time the clock says it is time to eat. It has been found that restrictive diets do not tend to work out most of the time as people tend to get so starved both physically and emotionally that when they are permitted to eat, they just go wild and opt for eating in order to fill the deprivation. Any kind of diet that keeps you preoccupied with the next meal is nothing more than a recipe to binge. You will have to ensure that you are not letting yourself stay hungry for a long period of time while being on intermittent fasting. Well, this can be easily achieved by opting for the right foods during the eating window.

Not Having Enough During The Eating Period

Not eating enough during the eating window can also lead to weight gain. Is it true? Well, yes, it is.

Besides having too many unhealthy food items during the eating window, not having enough food also cannibalizes muscle mass. All it leads to is slowing down your metabolism. Without the metabolic muscle mass, you might just sabotage your capability of burning fat in the future. The main challenge with intermittent fasting is that as you consume food according to some time-based rules in place of properly paying attention to the cues of the body, it is quite tough to know the actual needs. If you are making up your mind to give intermittent fasting a try, it is always suggested to consult a diet expert first who can help you assess and also meet the nutritional requirements with proper safety.

Ignoring "What" Because of "When"

Intermittent fasting is completely time-centered. The majority of the plans do not provide any kind of explicit rules regarding the types of food items that you need to during the eating window. However, that cannot be considered as an invitation to consume milkshakes, beer, French fries, and other unhealthy stuff. Fasting is not any kind of magic. Besides some small metabolic advantages, the primary impact on weight loss is mainly that you limit the eating hours. In short, you will have to limit the number of calories that you consume. However, the overall effect can be easily undone by opting for the wrong types of food items. You will have to make a shift from the perspective of 'treating yourself' mentality during the window of eating. Change the same to something that is mainly concerned about nutrient-dense foods. Try to make every meal of yours a proper combination of protein, fiber, and also healthy fats that will help you to get filled up and stay satisfied during the phase of fasting.

Chapter 13: Tips to Manage Menopause

The phase of menopause typically starts from the age of late 40s for the majority of women. Menopause tends to last for a few years. But the overall journey of the menopausal phase is not that smooth. It has been found that about 63.5% of women tend to suffer from the symptoms of menopause. Well, the symptoms seem to vary from one person to the other. Some of the common symptoms are:

- **Uncertainty of periods:** The early onset of menopause can be identified easily by uncertain or irregular periods.

- **Dryness:** Vaginal dryness is a very common menopausal symptom.

- **Night sweats:** Menopause might result in sweating during sleeping at night that tends to make sleep quite uncomfortable.

- **Mood swings:** Mood swings involve a sudden shifting of mood from good to bad and bad to good.

- **Weight gain:** Most women suffer from sudden weight gain at the time of menopause.

The uncertainty of the menstruation cycle varies from women to women. Generally, you will experience irregular periods right before they tend to end. Skipping of menstrual cycle at the time of menopause is quite a common and normal thing. Your menstruation cycle might just get skipped for a month or even more than that and then get back to normal after some months.

Having Enough Veggies and Fruits

When you try to include lots of veggies and fruits in your diet plan, you can easily get rid of the majority of the menopausal symptoms easily. Vegetables and fruits are low in calories and can also help you to stay full for longer time periods. So, by opting for veggies and fruits, you can easily lose excess body weight and also sustain the same. Fruits and vegetables are also great for the prevention of heart diseases as well. After the onset of menopause, the risk of developing heart diseases tends to increase. It is mainly because of the reduced levels of estrogen, gain in weight, and other factors. Also, consumption of vegetables and fruits will help you regain the lost bone strength.

Consumption of Enough Water

Dryness is a very common symptom that can be found during the onset of menopause. It is mainly the result of a reduction in the levels of estrogen. In order to deal with dryness, you will have to drink about ten to twelve glasses of water every day. It will also help in reducing the feeling of bloating that is quite common owing to the hormonal changes. Besides all of this, drinking plenty of water can also help in keeping a check on your weight gain. Water can keep you feel for a long time, and thus helping in weight loss. Adequate consumption of water also helps in enhancing the body's metabolism to a great extent. Also, drinking about 500 ml of water half an hour before the eating window can help in consuming about 14% lesser calories.

Having Food Items Rich In Calcium and Vitamin D

At the time of menopause, hormonal changes are bound to take place. It might lead to the weakening of bones. So, it can be said that menopause might also develop the chances of having osteoporosis. Whenever it is about proper health of bones, vitamin D and calcium just tops the list of essential nutrients. Including both these nutrients in your daily diet plan will help in regaining the lost bone strength, and having enough vitamin D-rich food items in your diet helps in cutting down the risk of fracturing your hip, as it is most likely to happen because of weak bones. Some of the most common calcium-rich food items are milk, yogurt, cheese, kale, collard greens, spinach, and many others. Also, you can find a high quantity of calcium in beans, sardines, and several other food items. In case you are not a great fan of veggies, shifting to calcium-fortified food items can also help, like several types of cereals, fruit juice, and milk alternatives.

Sunlight is often considered the greatest source of vitamin D. When your skin gets exposed to sunlight, vitamin D gets produced. But with growing age, the capability of the human skin to produce vitamin D directly from sunlight tends to reduce. In case you do not like to be under the sunlight for a long time, opting for supplements rich in vitamin D can also help. Cod liver oil, eggs, oily fish, and several other food items also act as great sources of vitamin D. So, in order to take care of your bone health, you will have to include enough vitamin D along with calcium in your daily diet.

Maintaining Healthy Body Weight

One of the most concerning symptoms of menopause is sudden weight gain. It generally results from alterations in hormones, lifestyle, genetics, and also aging. When the fat content of the body is quite high, specifically in the waistline area, the overall risk of developing serious health issues increases. You might even develop diabetes and chronic heart diseases. In fact, the general menopausal symptoms might get affected to a great extent because of weight gain. It has been found all those women who can discard about 18% - 22% of their body weight at the time of menopause can easily reduce the chances of having night sweats and hot flashes. So, maintaining a healthy weight is quite essential for dealing with menopausal symptoms.

Daily Workouts

There is a lack of evidence that can support whether exercising can help in dealing with night sweats and hot flashes. But can provide help in dealing with a range of other problems. Daily exercising will help you to enhance the rate of metabolism besides your levels of energy. Also, it helps in providing you with healthier bones and joints, better sleep, along with less stress.

According to a study, exercising for three hours every week for a year can help in the enhancement of mental as well as physical health. Besides that, it can improve the life quality of all those women who are going through the phase of menopause. Regularly working out also helps in the prevention of various diseases, such as heart diseases, type 2 diabetes, cancer, stroke, and obesity.

Keeping Distance From Trigger Foods

There are some food items that might act as triggers for various menopausal symptoms, like hot flashes, night sweat, and mood swings. When such food items are consumed during the nighttime, the symptoms might even get worse. Such food items include sugary items, alcohol, spicy food, and also caffeine. In order to find out which food items tend to act like a trigger to all your symptoms, you can maintain a journal for keeping a record of the symptoms. Whenever you think that some food items might be triggering your symptoms of menopause, opt for either reducing or stop having all such consumables. Maintaining your symptoms will be a lot easier if you can keep an eye on the trigger foods.

Consuming Food Items Rich In Protein

Consuming food items that come with a great amount of protein can help to preserve your muscle mass that you are most likely to lose because of aging. There is evidence that suggests that consumption of protein daily can help in slowing down the loss of muscles that is bound to happen from aging. Also, having food items rich in protein content can help in weight loss along with proper maintenance of lean muscles. In order to fulfill your daily dose of protein, you can have food items, like eggs, fish, meat, nuts, legumes, and dairy products. Just make sure that none of the food items act as a trigger for your symptoms.

Staying Away From Skipping Meals

Maintaining regular meals is quite important when you are going through the menopause phase. Trying to indulge in irregular eating patterns might just worsen the symptoms. Also, it might just hinder the efforts that you have already put into losing weight. Try to maintain your nutritional needs all the time so that you can easily reduce the symptoms related to menopause.

No Smoking

Smoking is not good for health, as we already know. It also increases the overall risk of osteoporosis, stroke, cancer, heart diseases, and many other chronic illnesses. It might also enhance the extent along with the severity of your hot flashes and night sweats. In fact, smoking continuously might lead to the early onset of the symptoms of menopause.

Having Food Items Rich In Phytoestrogen

Phytoestrogens are plant-based compounds that occur naturally. They provide great help in mimicking the overall effects of estrogen in the body of humans. So, consumption of the same can help in balancing the hormone levels. In Asian countries, like Japan, the consumption of this compound is quite high. That is the reason why women over there tend to suffer from very few hot flashes while being in the phase of menopause. There are several food items that come with this compound, like flaxseeds, soybeans, tofu, beans, tempeh, sesame seeds, and linseeds. However, the content of phytoestrogen in all these food items varies according to the methods of processing. If you try to follow a diet plan that comes packed with soy, it can help in the reduction of blood pressure, cholesterol, besides menopausal symptoms such as night sweats and hot flashes.

Staying Away From Processed and Refined Sugar Food Items

When you try to be on a diet plan which comes with high content of sugar and carbs, it might result in sharp falls and rises in the levels of blood sugar. So, it can easily make you feel irritated and tired. Opting for meals that are rich in carbs might also increase the chances of suffering from depression for all those women who just got done with the menopause phase. Diet plans composed of plenty of processed food can easily affect the health of your bones. In order to maintain your bone health, you will have to stay away from all kinds of processed food items and refined sugar.

Dealing With Symptoms

The symptoms of menopause might result in making your life quite troublesome. So, if you are willing to take care of the same, here are some tips for you.

Controlling night sweats

In order to deal with the problem of night sweats, you can opt for these strategies:

- Opt for sleeping in ultra-light clothes

- Have layered bedding so that it gets easier for you to remove the same at night

- Try to sleep with an extra electric fan right beside your bed

- Keep a jug full of cold water beside your bed at night so that you can have the same at regular intervals

- You can try to keep an ice pack underneath your pillow as it will help to cool you down; just flip the pillow after regular intervals for sleeping on a cooler surface

Urinary problems

While going through the phase of menopause, most women tend to suffer from bladder and urinary problems. It mainly results from the reduced levels of estrogen that ultimately leads to the weakening of the urethra muscles. In severe cases, menopausal women might find it hard to hold their urine for a long time right before going to the washroom. It is termed urinary urge incontinence. In fact, there are chances that the urine might just like if you try to cough, sneeze, or even laugh. It is termed urinary stress incontinence. In order to deal with all such problems in the most effective way, you can opt for certain medicines. Also, try to limit or even avoid consuming caffeine. The option that will fit you the best will completely depend on your overall condition. In case the condition keeps worsening, try taking the help of a doctor.

Anxiety and depression

While experiencing menopause, the chances are quite high that you suffer from anxiety and depression. It is primarily because of the hormonal changes. Also, you might experience sudden feelings of sadness as there might sudden changes in the levels of hormones in the body. Moreover, anxiety and depression can easily worsen your overall condition. Try to limit or avoid consumption of alcohol as it might dedicate to depression. Getting proper sleep might also help.

Mood swings

One of the most common symptoms of menopause is mood swings. You might get irritated or disturbed even with the smallest things. The best way in which this can be controlled is by keeping an active lifestyle. In case you are not much active in life, look out for ways so that you can be active on a daily basis. But ensure that you do not opt for a great number of duties at one time. Look out for some positive ways to ease your symptoms of stress.

If the symptoms of menopause tend to bother the natural course of your life, it will be better for you to opt for professional help. You will have to share the symptoms properly that you are facing.

Chapter 14: Exercises for Losing Weight

Besides dieting, exercising is one of the best strategies for shedding extra pounds. It helps in burning down calories and so plays an essential role in weight loss. Also, exercising helps in improving your overall mood, makes your bones stronger, and also reduces the risks of various chronic diseases. There are certain types of exercises that will readily help you lose weight besides opting for intermittent fasting or any other form of diet. Let's have a look at them.

Walking

Walking is often considered one of the best exercises for losing weight, and that is obviously for a good reason. It is an easy and convenient way for beginners to start working out without even getting overwhelmed or any need to buy equipment. In fact, walking is a kind of low-intensity excrcise, and so there will be less stress on your joints. It has been found that an individual of 70 kgs can burn about 166 calories for every 30 minutes of walking at a speed of 6.5 km/h. Also, a study involving twenty obese women found that walking for 40 – 7- minutes three times every week reduced their waist circumference along with body fat by approximately 1.2 inches and 1.4%, respectively. It is not a tough thing to include walking into your schedule.

For adding more steps to the course of your day, you can opt for walking during lunch break, opt for stairs instead of the elevator, or take your dog out for some walk. In order to get started with this, set a goal to walk for half an hour three to four times every week. As you get more fit, you can easily increase ten frequency and duration of your walks.

Running or Jogging

Running and jogging both are superb exercises for losing weight. Although both seem similar, the difference is that in jogging, you pace between 6.2 – 8.9 km/h, whereas, in the case of running, it is quite faster, like 9.8 km/h. It has been found that an individual of 70 kgs can burn about 297 calories for every half an hour jogging at a speed of 8 km/h, or 373 calories for every half an hour of running at a speed of 9.8 km/h. Also, studies revealed that running and jogging could help in burning down the harmful visceral fat, also known as belly fat. Belly fat wraps around the internal organs and is often linked to several chronic diseases, such as diabetes and heart disease. Both running and jogging are superb exercises that be performed anywhere and can also be included in your daily routine. In order to get started, set a goal of jogging for thirty minutes three to four times every week. In case you face difficulties in running or jogging outdoors, you can try running on soft surfaces, such as grass. You can also opt for treadmills that come with in-built cushioning, which might turn out to be easier on the joints.

Cycling

Cycling is quite a well-known exercise that helps in improving your level of fitness, besides helping you lose weight. Generally, cycling is done outdoors; however, many fitness centers and gyms come with stationary cycles that permit cycling while being indoors. It has been found that an individual of 70 kgs can burn about 263 calories for every half an hour of cycling on a stationary bike at a regular speed, or about 299 calories for every half an hour of cycling on a bicycle at a speed of 20 – 22.3 km/h. Besides assisting weight loss, cycling also helps in improving your overall fitness, lowers the risk of chronic heart conditions, and also increases sensitivity to insulin. Cycling can act as a great option for people of every fitness level, be it athletes or beginners. Also, cycling is a low-intensity exercise. So, there will be less stress on the joints.

Weight Training

Weight training is another choice that is available for all those people who are willing to lose weight. It has been found that you can burn about 113 calories for every half an hour of weight training. Weight training helps a lot in building strength besides promotion of muscle growth, which can very easily raise your RMR or resting metabolic rate – the number of calories that you can burn while being at rest. A six-month study showcased that doing ten minutes of weight training about three times every week can help in increasing the rate of metabolism by about 7.3% on average. Also, it has been found that the human body can burn more calories even after getting done with weight training exercises, in comparison to aerobic exercises.

Interval Training

Also known as HIIT or high-intensity interval training, it is a term that indicates short periods of intense exercises that get altered with several periods of recovery. Generally, HIIT lasts for about fifteen to thirteen minutes and can help in burning down a great number of calories. A study involving nine men found that HIIT helped in burning 26% - 30% more calories every minute in comparison to other sectors of exercising, like cycling, weight training, and treadmill running. So, it can be said that HIIT can help in burning down more calories while dedicating less time to exercises. Also, it has been found that HIIT helps in burning belly fat, which acts as the risk factor for a wide range of chronic diseases.

It is quite easy to be included in your daily routine of exercises. All that you will have to do is to select an exercise type, like jumping, running, cycling, along with your rest times and exercises. For instance, pedal as fast as you can on a cycle for about thirty seconds and then pedal at a slow pace for about two minutes. Try repeating the pattern for about fifteen to thirty minutes.

Swimming

Swimming is an easy and fun way of losing weight and getting in shape. It has been found that you can burn about 232 calories for every half an hour of swimming. The way you swim can actually affect the number of calories that you burn. For every half an hour, an individual of 70 kgs can burn 296 calories while doing the backstroke, 375 calories while doing breaststroke, 374 calories while treading water, and 408 calories while doing butterfly. Swimming can be a great option for reducing the percentage of body fat, improves overall flexibility, and also reduces the risk factors of heart diseases, such as high levels of blood triglycerides and cholesterol. It is a low-impact exercise that is quite easy on the joints. It makes swimming a great option for all those individuals who suffer from joint pain or injuries.

Chapter 15: Intermittent Fasting and Its Effects In Slowing Down Aging

Every one of us wants to look young, right? All of us want to possess glowing and youthful skin. No matter what kind of products or cosmetics you opt for, getting natural healthy, and glowing skin is nearly impossible. Having a healthy mind and body can help a lot in making us youthful. But we tend to ignore our health most of the time. The inner health condition easily gets reflected on our faces. The key to glowing and healthy skin is our metabolism. Everything that you feed your body with will get reflected on the skin.

Causes of Aging

Is it even possible to slow down the speed of aging without going through expensive operations or treatments or without using any kind of expensive skin products? Question of this nature is quite common, and the answer is yes. But before starting with the same, you will need to be aware of the aging process. Right now, the free radical theory is taken as the theory of aging. Free radicals are molecules that are unstable and rich in oxygen. The process of oxidation produces them. Antioxidants provide the needed help in neutralizing free radicals. In fact, they contribute to deal with pathogens as well. But at times, the overall number of free radicals just turns out to be excessive. It generally results from cigarette smoke, radiation, environmental pollutants, constipation, inflammation, and stress. In all such cases, the body's antioxidants fail to maintain the free radicals. As the free radicals are highly reactive, they tend to bond with the cells of the body.

All it results in is damage. When free radicals keep bonding, they tend to break the healthy tissues. It results in artery blockage, impaired memory, wrinkles, and other signs of aging.

Anti-Aging Properties of Intermittent Fasting

It has been found that limiting the consumption of calories can help in the promotion of longevity. The main reason behind this is that it can help in maintaining the youthful condition of the mitochondria. When the mitochondria remain in their youthful state, it is possible to establish better communication with the other parts of the cells. Such kind of communication is important for keeping up with various body functions. When mitochondria remain in one state, the effects of intermittent fasting can be focused on longevity. Because of this phenomenon, intermittent fasting is able to help in the prevention of aging. Indeed, there is no form of evidence till now for determining the actual reason behind this. But science is not conclusive all the time.

One of the best ways of restricting calorie intake is intermittent fasting. When the mitochondria are in the youthful state, we tend to live longer. So, it can be said that intermittent fasting provides us with several other benefits besides weight loss. Moreover, intermittent fasting helps in reducing inflammation besides reducing oxidative stress as well. But whether intermittent fasting can contribute to slowing down aging all the time is not known yet. However, being a healthy type of fasting, it can definitely help in maintaining a healthy lifestyle.

Intermittent Fasting and Skin Health

When you opt for fasting, the body remains without food for a long time. It also initiates several metabolic alterations in the body. The human body gets energy from the food that we eat. Whenever the food supply gets halted, the body starts depending on the stored body fats. Our body starts drawing the needed energy from the stored body fats by a process known as gluconeogenesis. The necessary glucose amount gets extracted by our body from various non-carbohydrate sources, like amino acids. When you start fasting, the pyrimidine and purine levels also tend to rise, which comes with some sort of direct effect on enhancing the antioxidant levels. When the level of antioxidants rises, the health of our body and skin also gets better. It also helps in the maintenance of balance between several body functions at the time of fasting.

It is the natural mechanism of the body that starts at the time of fasting. Also, it provides necessary help in filling up the losses that result from free radicals and oxidative stress. Intermittent fasting also initiates the process of autophagy that helps in throwing out all forms of waste from the cells. It can also be related to slowing down the process of aging as the metabolism of the body stays preserved for dealing with various types of cellular stress. So, it can be said that intermittent fasting can readily help in slowing down the aging process.

Conclusion

Thank you for making it through to the end of the *Intermittent Fasting for Women Over 50*; let's hope it was informative and able to provide you with all of the tools you need to achieve your goals, whatever they may be.

Intermittent fasting is not at all a complex thing. All you need to do is to dedicate some of your time to get hold of the same, and you can see the results in no time at all. Try to put into use the tips and strategies that you found in this book, specifically if you are over the age mark of 50. Right before you start, get proper knowledge about intermittent fasting from this book, and slowly pace the same. Just be patient and consistent with everything you do. Intermittent fasting cannot be compared to any other typical diet plan, and so it is easier to get started with as well.

You can keep consuming food of your choice. Just pay attention to maintain a healthy lifestyle and opt for nutrient-rich consumables. Maintain your fasts properly and try your best not to break the fast before the eating window. Do not rush yourself and start with a 24-hour fast straightaway. Include the recipes that you found in this book in your daily diet plan and fulfill the necessary nutrient requirements while fasting as well.

Finally, if you found this book useful in any way, a review on Amazon is always appreciated!

www.ingramcontent.com/pod-product-compliance
Lightning Source LLC
LaVergne TN
LVHW091550060526
838200LV00036B/781